Bangers and Mash

How to take on throat cancer, chemotherapy, radiotherapy and win, with help from an NLP coach.

Keith Hern

ISBN13 9781904312772

Published in the UK by
MX Publishing,
335, Princess Park Manor, Royal Drive, London, N11 3GX
www.mxpublishing.co.uk

This book is dedicated to Mel.

Contents

Timelines

This is not a complete list of the treatment, but hopefully provides a good insight into the timescales involved.

May 2007:

12th   first discovered the 'lump.'
15th   appointment at the GPs.
17th   ENT (ear, nose, throat) specialist – New Victoria Hospital.
23rd   ultrasound and biopsy – Parkside Hospital.
25th   diagnosis, consultant meeting at St.Anthony's Hospital.
30th   first NLP/coaching session.
31st   MRI scan – St. Anthony's.

June 2007:

1st   PET and CT scans – London medical centre.
5th   St Anthony's first operation to remove primary tumour.
7th   first consultant meeting at The Royal Marsden.
8th   coaching session.
18th   EDTA pre-chemo kidney tests at The Marsden.
19-24th five day chemotherapy treatment – The Marsden.

July 2007:

4th   Coaching session.
11th   EDTA pre-chemo kidney tests at The Marsden.
12-18th five day chemotherapy treatment – The Marsden.
19th   MRI scan.
20-29th escape to Elba and Tuscany!
30th   radiotherapy planning – The Marsden.
        CT scans with radiotherapy mask.

August 2007:

6th   start of daily radiotherapy at The Marsden each day for six weeks.

9th   top-up chemotherapy session, overnight at The Marsden.

14th   CT scan – clinical trial.

20th   CT scan – clinical trial.

25th   bank holiday weekend away in Scotland.

28th   CT scan – clinical trial.

29th   coaching session.

September 2007:

Daily radiotherapy.

4th   CT scan – clinical trial.

6th   second chemo top-up overnight at The Marsden.

13th   final radiotherapy session. Check-up.

22nd   coaching session.

24th   'The Turning Point'.

27th   post radiotherapy check-up, The Marsden.

October 2007:

11th   next check-up The Marsden.

18th   MRI/CT/PET scan.

19-22nd   Italy trip.

November 2007:

1st   post-scan consultant check-up and review.

14th   pre-op check-up – Parkside.

20-22nd   second operation – St Anthony's.

30th   post-op check-up. End of treatment!

1. The Turning Point

The CornerHOUSE

Four months of treatment, medication, side effects, side effects of side effects, drugs, chemicals, scans, tests, and I'm sitting in Marney's, a picturesque local pub by a pond on Weston Green. I'm with two friends who have been kind enough to help me set up my photo exhibition starting tomorrow at The CornerHOUSE in Surbiton.

The menu's passed around, but in keeping with recent times, I order yet another bowl of soup, and yet another glass of water, and watch with slight envy as my mates tuck into platefuls of 'real food'.

Only this time it feels different: no real reason, can't explain why, but it just does.

'Can I try a mouthful?' I ask hesitantly.

'Go ahead' they say in stereo. 'Okay, I'll go for a spoonful of bangers and mash, with heaps of gravy'. They know what I've been through and that I haven't had solid food for weeks, so watch silently, waiting.

It must be awful to watch – a few mouthfuls of water with each small nibble, a much laboured chew and an awkward swallow. It seemed to take for ever.

'And another please' I ask, surprising myself 'and another'.

It's not easy, but I want to keep going. Maybe, just maybe? After all this time. I've got some solid food down. Is this it? Have I finally reached the turning point? I do believe I have. At last, after all this time, I really believe this is it. I'm on the mend!'

It's impossible to describe just how good this felt. I can't taste anything yet, but I can get solid food down again, albeit in very small amounts. The months of treatment suddenly seem like a bad dream – I'm quietly ecstatic.

It's Monday 24th September 2007 – eleven days after the last bout of radiotherapy, and the first small (or should that be large?) step forward. 'No more detours' as Helen would say!

I get home, and can't wait to see the girls and impart my news. *'So you managed a couple of mouthfuls of bangers and mash, big deal'* I can almost hear Jess saying. But not a bit of it, they were every bit as delighted as I was.

Photo exhibition

Now for a small matter of my photo exhibition which is starting tomorrow evening – running for five nights in tandem with the 'soon-to-be-famous-One-Acts' at the CornerHOUSE. As I've exhibited there before, and Jess (my daughter) has been in various plays, the regulars are up to speed with what's been going on in my life.

Real life

'Will anyone turn up?' I wonder as I prepare for the private view.

I've sent out loads of invitations, had it promoted in the local press and on local radio. So now the acid test. Will anyone turn up? Will I sell anything?

Having had a few months of pretty much zero earnings the business now needs to start moving. Earning some money again would be useful - I'm sure Mads (my wife) would agree!

The nervous wait is always the same, but I needn't have worried - over a hundred people turn up.

Everyone politely comments on 'how well you're looking'. *'Hardly'* I think, as there are bones sticking out of my body I never knew existed, my trousers are virtually falling off as my waist has shrunk so much, I'm white as a sheet, and my face looks like an extra from an old horror movie with skin almost falling off the bones. But, who cares? I've just taken my first steps on the road to recovery.

This was the first opportunity I had had to introduce Mads to Helen, and I wanted them to meet, as I firmly believe the therapeutic coaching work done with Helen has been a massively important factor in me getting this far.

'Mads meet Helen'. To say I was totally unprepared for what happened next would be a massive understatement. Mads, normally the picture of self-control and tower of mental strength, just burst into tears.

In case there had been any shred of doubt this just confirmed: firstly, exactly how much help Helen had been, and secondly, the unbelievable stress Mads and Jess had been living under the last few months. How Mads has managed to keep working and remain outwardly calm I just can't begin to comprehend, but just count myself very lucky to have two such strong ladies at home.

The evening is going very well, a good atmosphere, loads of people (I don't even have time to say more than hi to most of them), decent weather, plenty of wine being drunk, and even the occasional passing remark along the lines of 'good photos'.

After everything that I've been through my recurring thought is *'it's just fantastic to be alive, be here and be on the mend'*.

With the 10.30 finish looming there's suddenly a rush of people eager to part with their money and buy the photos – I knew that investment in free wine would work! I end up taking over £1000 of orders, way beyond my expectations.

Time for just one more celebratory 'mineral water'.

Half pint

The hockey season is starting - Jess plays matches on a Sunday, and trains on a midweek evening, along with a few of her school mates.

The midweek training session has become a bit of a social as the small, but very select, group of taxi-driving Dads use it as a great excuse for a quiet social drink when the girls are training.

This Sunday turns out to be different: the match has been cancelled, so another training session has been arranged and all the 'drivers' are present. It's one of those warm, sunny September days, the sort that should be here throughout the summer, but somehow didn't quite make it this year.

Finishing training the girls were hot and thirsty, and one of them asks for a drink. 'May as well join them?' someone suggests.

'This could be interesting, what will this taste like?' Knowing my usual taste another Dad asks: 'Pint of London Pride as usual Keith?'

'I'll try a half', my first alcoholic drink in nearly two months. It duly arrives, conversation slows and I can feel all these eyes watching me to see what's going to happen. Here goes - the first mouthful.

'How grim is that!'

There will obviously need to be some practice as it's only three weeks until I go to Tuscany with Mads. By then I must be able to eat cheese and meat and manage a glass of red – or two perhaps. First things first – another check-up to go through....

That familiar trip

Mads comes up to the Marsden Hospital with me for the next check-up.

After the usual wait it's in to see Andrew Jones, my consultant for chemo and radiotherapy. He feels my neck, sticks 'that' camera up my nose and down my throat. Mads grimaces and turns away. She never has been able to watch this particular test.

Next he dons this strange reflective round metal device with a hole in it to peer into my mouth, and calls Mads over to have a look. The yellow gunk in the back of my mouth has started reducing, and the strawberry effect on the roof of my mouth is starting to recede. All is going well he assures us.

Still, I will have to wait a while until the result of the treatment is known. That won't be until the effect of the radiotherapy has died down a bit, so it will be another few weeks, probably late November, before I know what the prognosis is. Anyway, needless to say there is a holiday planned to get over all the treatment - *'focus on the destination, not the detours.'*

Helen's words never seem far away – how often have I needed them over the past few months?

Now, it's time for the all-important question to Andrew about the family Christmas trip to recuperate. Even by our adventurous standards this holiday will be something special. One night in Johannesburg, five nights on La Reunion, nine nights in Madagascar and finish off with five nights in Sun City and a Soweto tour on the way back to the airport. Should be a very special trip, and ideal r&r for what has been one grim year.

The rather large final bill for the trip is at home so this is it.

'Am I okay to go Andrew?' I blurt out, all pretence at subtlety completely out of the window.

Andrew gives me one of those 'knowing looks' and smiles. 'Tuscany in July, Tuscany in a couple of weeks, and now this?' he replies, then pauses.

'Yes you can go. Even if the end-of-treatment prognosis is bad you can go, and then re-start treatment after getting back'. Fantastic news.

It occurs to me that there could be an interesting conversation with the travel insurance company about cover and 'pre-existing conditions'.

Meat and red wine

Tuscany is looming large now - I've tried a few glasses of wine and some Italian food but the taste buds aren't great, chewing is still difficult. However there are the first signs that things are starting to improve.

Also, the side effects of the treatment have started to calm down. I still have a permanently dry mouth so am always sipping at water, but that could last for ages. I am starting to be able to eat more in the way of solids again, and even manage a glass of wine or two: '*Training for Tuscany*'.

I've started putting weight back on, and quite quickly as well, but there is a long way to go to turn this skeleton back into its previously impressive 'thirteen stone weakling' frame.

What I have noticed on the odd not-so-warm day is how chilly it is around the back of my neck, but I'm obviously starting to get my strength back as I can now hit a golf ball at least one hundred and fifty yards, so it's coming together.

Italy

It's the 19th October, some five weeks after my last radiotherapy session, and departure date to Tuscany. Jess decided ages ago that with no swimming pool and no mates she'd rather stay at home than go to Italy with the 'old farts'. She has a good, healthy teenage attitude now, which is great, and leaves us to spend three days wining and dining, and, well, wining and dining.

'Have I done sufficient training for this?' Even though the appetite is still small and the taste limited, the food is just so good there I'm sure it'll be fine. We have a fantastic time, and true to form, manage to over-indulge in spite of the treatment, and it felt great.

'We'll have to put you on withdrawal symptom watch then!' echoed round my head. It just seems so long ago that I heard that remark from the doctor.

We had been advised to go wine-tasting at Montalchino, which turned out to be fabulous. Numerous full-bodied Brunellos, and some 'prosciutto e formaggio' (which somehow always sounds so much tastier than ham and cheese!). It takes for ever to chew, but there is just a further hint that the taste buds are awakening – sure the Brunello helps!

On our first night we headed straight for our newly-found favourite restaurant: 'La Vecchia Banana' in Pondetera, owned by a fabulous chef and his wife who have run restaurants in the middle east, Thailand and Taiwan to name but a few.

The meal was so good, that on our last day we just about had time to visit them again. One small problem was that we needed to be in and eating before their normal opening time in order to catch the plane home.

Trying our luck we rang and they agreed to open early especially for us. *'I wonder what the chances would be of a restaurant back home being so accommodating?'* What a great way to end an excellent three days. Accompanied by another fine bottle of 'Scarlet', from the vineyard down the road at Peccioli – after all it was their tip to visit the restaurant in the first place – one more superb meal, a couple of 'arrivedercis' and it was off to the airport.

We even made some rash promise to learn some Italian before coming again – one glass of Scarlet too many? Linguistically I'm a typical Brit, and don't speak any other language. Mads, however, as well as her native Swedish and English is also fluent in German, Danish and Norwegian and understands a lot of French and Dutch. It's so impressive, not to mention useful, to be able to swap between languages so casually. Eight months until we plan to be back in Tuscany– get learning!

In the meantime it's back home. **THE** all-important check-up is now looming large.

2. How It All Began

Kitchen chat

It was mid-afternoon on a sunny Saturday in May; I'd just got back from playing golf and was chatting with Mads in the kitchen. Nothing important, just the usual husband and wife conversation about the weekend plans, what Jess was up to, the weekend shopping – normal family conversation.

I leant my head back, and rubbed my neck – no apparent reason, just did it. There seemed something a little unusual on the left side of my neck. Mads saw my reaction and enquired 'what is it?'

'Don't know' I replied, 'you know when you get a cold and the glands in your neck swell up, well it's a bit like that, but only on one side – the left.'

'Does it hurt?'

'No, not at all, in fact it's so small I can hardly feel it'.

'You better get it checked out just to be safe', she advised.

Within a couple of days I was at the doctor's. First the junior doctor took a look, then the senior doctor. Both agreed – they don't think it's anything to worry about, but want me to go and get a second opinion from an ENT (ear, nose and throat) specialist.

The next stop was hospital, and the ENT specialist had another look around and basically repeated what the doctor had said, 'I'm 95% sure there's nothing wrong, but would like you to go for a biopsy just to be sure. We'll arrange a meeting in a couple of weeks to go through the test results.'

Fine with me.

The call

Thinking back I wonder what that morning was like for him. I imagine him breakfasting as usual – probably the healthy option of fruit juice, some prunes and maybe a sprinkling of bran and mint tea. Maybe the mint was from the garden, making it all the better.

I think of him taking his time – knowing that breakfast was the highlight of a day that probably wouldn't improve until he returns home at 7pm to a much needed G&T. My God he must need those sometimes, after what he has to do on days like this.

He is probably restricting himself to a couple of glasses of wine with dinner nowadays. Merlot – I bet that's his favourite, although no doubt he pays attention to the alcohol percentages on the back in deference to the ticker.

I think he is pretty happy in his work most of the time. He's made good progress up through the ranks and is highly thought of by his peers. He's made it and, most days, he must get satisfaction with being able to dispense healing or, at the very least, minimise the pain of patients in his care.

But even after all these years in his job, I'll bet he never gets used to what he has to do today. This must be the worst part by far and dealing with it is something that's impossible to teach at medical school.

Four calls to make this morning and they would be all over by midday.

He's an empathetic man – he won't be good for anything in the afternoon. Administrative work only for the rest of day. Perhaps he found time to get that paper finished for the conference where he was the keynote speaker.

I see him preoccupied, distracted and uncomfortable as he eases his 7 series BMW out of the gravel driveway.

The call

This time will be etched on my mind forever. It was 11.15 on the morning of Friday 25th May 2007.

I was busy processing the latest batch of shots on the computer, just waiting for my 11.30 visitor to turn up. I was munching on a couple of rounds of toast smeared with perhaps too much marmite, even for me. Madeleine wouldn't let me near her for at least an hour after my elevenses.

It had been a tricky shoot, the weather had been against me and the client needed the usual massaging but I knew I'd pulled it out of the bag. Making the decision to career swap and go freelance was the best thing I had ever done.

I answered the mobile when it rang. *'That's all I need,'* I thought, *'the client's going to be late'.*

I recognised the distinctive voice at the other end immediately.

'Mr. Hern, the results of your tests are in,' said the consultant with no preamble. 'We'd like you to go to St. Anthony's in Cheam to see a consultant called Mr. Timothy at 1.30 this afternoon.'

'I'm sorry, I've got a visitor turning up in fifteen minutes who will have driven an hour to get here, can we make it later in the day?'

'Mr. Hern,' he said firmly, 'You need to go and see him at 1.30.'

It was as if I was allowed no questions or alternatives, and he could at least have called me Keith.

'Okay, I'll ring my client and tell him I can't make the meeting.'

In a daze, I made the call straight away. I intimated I'd had some bad news, and ended the conversation abruptly.

It was only when I put the phone down did it dawn on me exactly what the consultant had *'really'* just said.

The tests had been done two weeks previously. We had arranged I would go back for a post-test assessment meeting on 5th June, but that I would call on Tuesday 29th May, just to check whether there was anything sinister going on. This was four days early – the nerve-ends started jangling at the realisation of what that meant.

What he had left unsaid was the real message, which was clearly, 'those tests on that innocuous-feeling small lump on your neck have returned positive. YOU HAVE CANCER!'

The realisation dawned, the emotions kicked in and, like a small child who had been hurt, suddenly gripped by fear, I just sat there and broke down in an uncontrollable flood of tears.

The psychic fly on the wall would have heard my now-racing thoughts, and rapidly gathering mental turmoil.

'How serious is it?'
'Will I survive?'
'What about my Jess?'
'And poor Mads?'
'How will they cope?'
'Shit! Shit! Shit!'
'Why me?'
'What have I done to deserve this?'

19

'I'm too young to die'.

Then a brief practical thought appeared from nowhere.

'Madeleine lands at 12.45.'
'Jess will want her lunch at 1.30. Bloody school closing a half day on Fridays. What's the government playing at? She'll have to sort herself out. Must leave a note'.
'The bloody car'.

I will have to get a move on to make that 1.30 appointment at the hospital.

I'd only dropped the car off at the dealer around the corner to trade it up, that morning. I had to come back car-less because the bank couldn't authorise payment for the new one. I needed a car to get to Cheam so I shut down the pc, wiped a few more tears away, wrote a quick note for Jess and left in a hurry.

It was only as the door slammed behind me that I checked I'd got my keys, and wallet. *'Thank Christ, stop falling apart, and hold yourself together'.*

I'd failed to notice it was raining. The fine sort of English 'mizzle' that was harder than drizzle, but not quite rain. Getting wet was the least of my worries. My mind was in freefall now, and all over the place.

'Must mend that fence when I get back'
'The Irish called it a soft day'.
'That tile is going to fall off the roof and hurt someone if he doesn't fix it'.

Craig the new neighbour was really letting his house go. *'Why are all these thoughts entering my head? I've just been told I've got cancer!'*

As I was walking to the dealers I was sure I could hear. *'Ha ha, ha ha, we're those little cancer cells and we've got you now. Ha ha, ha ha.'* (I was in the middle of reading Stephen King's 'The Tommyknockers'.)

When I got there the salesman wasn't around to do the deal. I negotiated the keys back for the old car.

I didn't have a hands-free so I called Mads' number from the dealer's forecourt – thought it was better she got some kind of message.

'What if her plane was late? Or early? Or she got home to find I wasn't there?'

Shaking I dialled, obviously she's not landed, the messaging service is on. 'Hi love it's me, the test results are in. It's serious, I'm off to see a consultant called Mr. Timothy right now – it's about 12.45'. That was all I could blurt out before being overcome again.

She had been on a five-day business trip to India. This was not the sort of news anyone wanted to hear when they get back.

It was only then I touched my neck – the lump was tiny. Surely something this small couldn't kill me? A shiver went down my spine at the thought; goose-bumps appeared up both my arms. My mind was all over the place.

'There's no way I'm going to be able to take Jess to Devon'.
'Maybe I should cancel the new car? But they've got my money.'
'Will I ever be able to lead Jess down the aisle now?'
'Ha ha, ha ha, got you!'

I got to St. Anthony's in plenty of time. God knows how I didn't have an accident. Couldn't think straight. Can't even remember the journey. I parked right outside – just as well as the rain hadn't eased at all.

As I got out the car there was a message from Mads on the mobile.

'Where are you? What's happened?' Oh God, I hadn't left any information on where I was going or anything!

Managed to reach her and just managed to tell her about 'The Call' and where I was now. Needless to say my message had put her in a real state.

'I'll be back around 2.30. No point in you coming over. We'll know more then.'

I headed for the hospital entrance. The sliding doors opened for me, then closed behind me. I felt like I'd just been beamed up into a whole new world.

At least I didn't have to wait long. On the dot of 1.30 I met Mr. Timothy. I guessed they kept to time by keeping extraneous dialogue to an absolute minimum, with no doubt a queue of patients to be seen after me.

'Come in Mr. Hern,' he said and, at least, shook my hand.

Without taking so much as a breath after he sat down, he said, 'Right, the test results have shown the lump in your neck to be cancerous'.

'This is for real'

'So just to absolutely clarify' I said remarkably calmly, 'I have cancer?'

'Yes' he replied, delivering the final knock-out blow.

The aftermath

The drive back was even more of a haze than the drive there.

Jess was in front of the TV. 'Mum's in the bath,' she said without looking up.

'She doesn't know'.

I walked into the bathroom, 'I'm scared', was all I could muster, 'welcome home' seeming somewhat academic.

As Mads got out of the bath, normally the epitome of self-control, even she lost all composure and we embraced, now in floods of tears – not bothered how wet my clothes were getting. After a while I got her a towel and said 'I need to tell Jess'.

As I came back into the living room, I could see she was now pretending to do homework. She must have instinctively known something was up as the TV was off.

Sitting down beside her on the settee, I took her hand, and looking into those beautiful blue eyes, started. My eyes were welling up.

'Jess darling, the test results are in – I've got cancer'.

A look of terror overcame her pretty little face; she screamed hysterically and flung her arms around me.

Another tearful embrace 'Are you going to die Dad?'

'We'll get through it, but we all need to be strong and positive' I mumbled, totally unsure where that came from.

The tears began to subside, Madeleine appeared and as a family we just sat hugging each other while I mustered the composure to talk through the day's events.

'After he confirmed it was indeed cancer, he put one of those funny little cameras at the end of a thin tube up one of my nostrils'. What a weird sensation that is, especially when you can feel it going down into the throat! I am going to have to get used to this.

'So what is the next step?' asked Mads.

'How did they know it's cancer?' interjected Jess.

I explained the meetings at the GPs, the specialist at the New Victoria and then the biopsy at Parkside Hospital. 'What's a biopsy?' asked Jess.

'I had the 'bump' lanced and they took a sample away for analysis'.

'Yuk, sounds lovely, not!' said Jess.

'Next it's back to Mr Timothy at St Anthony's, then the Marsden for more tests and to plan the chemotherapy and radiotherapy treatment in detail, then various types of scans – CT, MRI and PET.' The start date is June 5th when it's into St Anthony's for various tests and the first operation.'

Mr Timothy had explained 'that's the time to remove the offending primary tumour on the back of your tongue, and I will probably whip out the tonsils at the same time.'

'Then we need to wait until the scan results are known, probably start the chemo at The Marsden in mid-June for a week.'

'What about work?'

'Not sure right now. I'll be home for two weeks after that before going back in for another week of chemo, then a break, and then the radiotherapy starts. No idea how I'll feel but may be able to slot something in, who knows maybe I'll manage a shoot or two, but if not I'll just work on the website and start planning for the exhibition later this year.'

I was pretty sure I wouldn't be up to either, but now was not the time to show it, so a brave face was the order of the day.

'Let's get the car' I suggested and we headed up to the garage.

'You okay? I hear you had to go out in the old car while I was out,' said the rather portly salesman. *'Why did they all wear those anoraky jackets? It makes him look twice the size.'*

'Had a bit of an urgent issue to attend to, I had to go to hospital as I've just been diagnosed with cancer,' I said rather matter-of-factly, as if it happened every day. It was just over four hours since 'The Call'.

It transpired his wife had survived a horrendous bout of breast cancer.

'If my wife's experiences were anything to go by you'll soon be able to write a guide to hospitals you've known and loved in the South of England'.

'Great. I wonder if you can accrue medical air miles?'

Driving rather gingerly we made the two-minute drive home, and the mood had picked up – whether it was the new car, or the knowledge that other people get cancer and survive, I don't know. The girls are ready so we take the new car for a spin and visit a pub in Ockham I haven't been to for probably twenty five years.

Strangely the mood is quite positive, we have a nice drink, I play a couple of games of pool with Jess. I let her win the first, but get beaten fair and square in the next. To anyone

25

watching we look like a normal family, without a care in the world.

Back home and I cooked a really nice pasta al Fredo – a calorie-heavy sauce made from butter, cream and parmesan cheese, but a favourite of mine and Jess. I opened a nice bottle of Chianti to wash it down.

We even let Jess have half a glass. Without prompting, or the usual groan, she volunteered to clear up, loaded the dishwasher then came to give me a big hug before going to bed.

We weren't far behind her.

I swore I heard '*ha ha, ha ha.*'

Life goes on......

In amongst the mental mayhem from the new medical 'issue' I'd received two bits of excellent news about my photography. Oh yes, I will still need to keep in touch, and if possible earn some money in the months to come.

Timesonline had emailed me to confirm they were going to use my Kenyan photos in their 'travel photographer portfolio' feature in the next couple of weeks, something I'd been working on for quite a while.

Out of the blue the Daily Mail had rung about some of my Italian shots they'd found on one of the photo libraries I supply images to. They were going to run an article on a German developer who had bought up swathes of prime Tuscan countryside for a major holiday development, and I happened to have some landscape shots taken around Castelfalfi, precisely where the development was planned.

It will be interesting to see what happens with both of these.

As a regular on the local business networking circuit, at one recent meeting I had met, and had a brief chat with Helen, an experienced professional coach and NLP (Neuro Linguistic Programming) trainer.

'Don't suppose you do some sports psychology?' I'd enquired in an offhand manner, having been struggling with that most frustrating of sports, golf.

'Sure,' she replied, so duly booked the free initial half hour chat. To say things had changed since that initial meeting would be an understatement, so emailed something along the following lines:

'Hi Helen can we keep the 30 minutes but move it earlier in the day, oh and a minor change to the subject matter – I've just been diagnosed with cancer!'

The response was almost immediate, 'bollocks to the thirty minutes, you've got an initial three hour session, ring me and let's start' she emailed back. What a perfect response! For the first time in four hours I laughed - what a great feeling. How very strange to notice.

I knew my mind had been all over the place, but this was something else – noticing such strange little things. What a coincidence meeting her.

'No such thing as coincidence' she would advise me in due course!

Sleeping wasn't easy, in fact I spent half the night awake. *What the hell is going to happen to me? What is the treatment going to be like? Will I survive, or is this it?*

After this somewhat restless night it was off to play golf on Saturday morning.

'How will I cope with seeing loads of old friends with my latest piece of news?'

One of the guys I was playing with had gone through exactly the same scenario last year. I'd spoken to him briefly yesterday afternoon, and he'd invited Madeleine and I round later to discuss the fun-and-games heading in my direction, and also give some (invaluable) input as to how to cope from the partners' side.

Concentration on golf isn't great (wonder why?), but all in all, I'm fairly proud of myself for keeping (okay, almost keeping) control. Got back home about two to find the girls had been out for some retail therapy, and the mood was good, although Jess was complaining about stomach pain.

Jess seemed okay so we headed off to see Robin and Chris to find out what was in store for me. His cancer experience started in an almost identical way to mine: small lump in the neck, no real pain, better get it checked out, GP, hospital, poking and prodding, biopsy, blood tests, op and into the chemo and radiotherapy. Chris, his wife, it seems, is very similar to Mads in attitude – instead of just accepting what the 'experts' tell you, it's: 'Why?' 'How?' 'When?' 'So what?' etc…

Chris said the first key point as far as she was concerned was the surgery, knowing the lump had been removed, followed up quickly by the scan results as it proved that the throat lump was a solitary tumour in Robin's case.

Medical advice from one of experience: get both CAT and PET scans. It sounded more like some vet's practice than cancer treatment! The PET scan apparently is vital as it involves being pumped full of radioactive glucose, to which any active cancer cells react so can be easily identified, thereby confirming the extent of any cancer.

Robin said he couldn't believe that I was already talking so much about the situation and keeping control. *'Not so sure about the control part!'*

I even discovered what chemotherapy actually involves, not having been that bothered previously. It sounds like some kind of rather unpleasant experiment from the science lab.

After all, cancer, like other serious illnesses, only ever happens to other people. This is already somewhat of a wake-up call to my own mortality, not to say vulnerability.

Phone call

Suddenly the mobile rang.

It was Jess in floods of tears saying how her stomach was really painful, so we made a quick dash home – what a great Bank Holiday weekend this is turning out to be!

Off to A&E. The staff at the hospital, as ever, were first rate (Jess had previously been in for meningitis as a baby and nephrotic syndrome, a kidney disorder, twice when a little younger). After a couple of hours, some poking and prodding she was admitted for overnight observation and almost certain surgery in the morning –appendix removal.

I stayed with her - dozing off in hospital….

'Was that a headache behind the left ear?'
'Why is the bottom of my back giving me gyp?'
'Was that mole really there?'
'Go to SLEEP!'

'Oh Helen, do you know what you're about to take on!'

Saw the surgeon, the op went fine and Jess is recovering.

Back home the phone went and it was Madeleine's father. Explained that Jess was in hospital, but didn't know the Swedish for appendix, so left a message for Madeleine to call, and also ducked my situation.

Time for night shift again so back to the hospital to keep Jess company. Her spirits are picking up now as the post-op blurriness subsides. I just look at her lying in the hospital bed: '*God she's so beautiful; I love her so much!*'

I was pretty knackered and, try as I might, couldn't stay awake so fell asleep first. 'Situation normal,' she observed the following morning. (I have a reputation at home for an unerring ability to doze off in front of the TV, regardless of how 'interested' I am in whatever I was watching.)

Woke up with a start in a cold sweat in the middle of the night - I'd been dreaming and had just been present at my own wake. God that was creepy – '*what is this cancer doing to my head already?*'

Jess is recovering – she's in good spirits after her hospitalisation experience.

My turn next!

Heard the news?

Madeleine's just appeared for the next hospital shift, and we wander off for a coffee. She managed to tell her parents the news and kept control, although did admit to shedding a few tears in private. Her boss rings while we're out and says he'll cover for her when necessary over the next few weeks. Nice of him.

We have no real idea about what's coming – the unknown is very scary!

We held hands tightly; both scared.

Emotions are running like a rollercoaster at the moment. Even just writing down what I'm going through brings a lump in my throat. The only time I've ever been through anything like this on the mental front was when Jess was six months old, and we were in exactly the same place as we are now – Kingston Hospital.

That started on a Friday as well, and she had been in the children's ward all week for tests, no results. The ward had been cleared when we arrived. Baby Jess had been taken for a lumber puncture and we were told she had meningitis. The word no parent wants to hear. 'What's the bottom line?' I had asked nervously, wanting a straight answer. As if reading my mood he calmly stated 'okay, if she's here on Monday she'll live'.

I won't ever forget that weekend. Needless to say she pulled through. Now let's work on ensuring my outcome is as successful.

'How am I going to play this?'

I'm off to see my family down in Sussex and will have to tell them, and am not looking forward to this at all. After a very nerve-racking drive down to Sussex, I arrive surprised at how calm I am. Fortunately it is just my parents.

Mentally I had gone through numerous ways as to how to handle the situation, eventually deciding this couldn't be overly planned, so fell back on 25 years of sales experience and relied on the tried and tested formula 'If in doubt, blag it!'

All was going okay until just one question too many about why I hadn't rung to say the girls weren't coming.

'This is it...'

31

'Okay, I have something to tell you. A few weeks ago I found a small lump in my neck, and have been for various hospital visits and tests. The results came through on Friday and I have throat cancer!'

Not easy to tell them, and while Dad was the picture of control, Mum and I shared a tearful hug. Dad was the epitome of a stoic Englishman, displaying a supreme stiff upper lip, just nodded acknowledgement and said 'okay'.

'Okay? Okay? What do you mean okay?'

Not sure I could react that way if Jess had just dropped a bombshell like this! All in all it went better than I had expected, so set off for home in good spirits, and had a much more relaxed drive back.

The mobile rang. 'Can you pick up Jess' hairbrush on your way into hospital?' She's obviously fine!

Leaving Jess in hospital for one last night Madeleine and I took the chance to go out to a restaurant for a 'normal' evening, and picked 'Sherpa's Kitchen', an excellent Nepalese restaurant in Esher. A group of four sat at the next table, one of whom I'd last seen only a few days ago on the real tennis court – small world!

'How are you?'

'Now there's a question!'

'Where shall I start?' 'Great, I've just been diagnosed with cancer' were answers that sprung to mind, but opted for the more straightforward 'fine'. An old pro at handling this already. Anyway, excellent food as ever: nice and spicy, but not too hot, strong flavours, not too filling like many a curry – all in all a very enjoyable evening.

Can't help but wonder when will I next be eating spicy food? Rumours of the side effects of what I'm about to go through are starting.

Now to focus on work – almost forgotten about that. I'm doing a shoot for one of my biggest customers in a truly exotic location - a pub in Camberwell. As ever with this customer the shoot is entertaining and always slightly different to what is expected beforehand.

Successfully completed, I headed back confident in the knowledge that the house would soon be alive with teenagers coming to view Jess' scar!

Taxi service

'How's the patient?' asked one of the drivers (i.e. parent).

'Would that be young or old?' I replied.

Word had spread about my diagnosis, but not to everyone apparently, as she looked positively shell-shocked when I told her. Another parent appeared a while later to collect a couple of the kids, and wanted some clarification of a passing comment her daughter had made, in that wonderfully nonchalant way that kids have.

'I think Keith's not well, cancer or something' was how she had dropped it into the conversation. So, I put her straight, and she stayed a while for a glass of wine and chatted through what was involved.

'How will this work moving forward?' I wonder.

Mental progress?

I'm starting to calm down a little now, as the acceptance of having got cancer has settled, and now it's 'just' a matter of working out how best to beat the disease.

Off to see a mate, and while en route get a call from a very old friend who had only just heard my news. I struggle with my emotions to go through what was going on but managed a quick chat. Moved ten yards along the road in another seemingly endless suburban traffic jam, then the message alert on the mobile went off.

Jess had sent the simple text message 'Dad I love you.' Too much for the current mental state, I just broke down in tears then and there. I've never experienced quite these levels of emotion before. So much for 'starting to calm down'.

Perhaps this NLP stuff will help – now is the time to find out.

Set off to see Helen, with absolutely not the faintest idea as to how she would approach helping me, nor, come to think of it, what was going to happen next.

'Hi Keith, come on in' she said in that very friendly way of hers.

Two hours plus of conversation without any mention of cancer. Just lots of questions, listening intently to my answers, querying here and there and generally building up a picture of what I am like as a person. A bit like what I would imagine lying on a psychiatrist's couch must be like. A little nerve-racking, as I could feel myself being gently eased out of my comfort zone, with some very carefully considered questions.

I would summarise my first NLP experience as strangely therapeutic, not always comfortable, and very thought provoking. Knowing hospital was approaching she had lent me a self-hypnosis CD to listen to. 'Preparing for a Medical Intervention' by Suzi Smith.

'What an intriguing title' I thought, putting it into the CD player in the car. The first words being 'don't listen to this in the car'. The temptation was to ignore this instruction, but concluded as it's designed to send you into some kind of hypnotic state, it would probably be safer for all other road users if I heeded the advice and waited until I was at home.

Walked in the front door, straight to the CD player and on with the hypnosis. It began with calming music (which reminded me of some meditative music heard at a remote religious festival many years ago on a back-packing trip in the Far East), followed by an extremely controlled voice. The essence of the message was simple – prepare yourself properly mentally and you'll be fine. So easy to say! Much to my surprise it was easy to follow and made sense. In my semi-trance the questions began:

- *do you know why you're undergoing a 'medical intervention'?*
- *what are the stages of the treatment and where do you want to be at the end of each stage?*
- *'transport' yourself to where the intervention is going to happen, look around – are you happy you have the right support?*
- *do those carrying out the intervention fill you with confidence?*
- *keep mindful of the desired outcome of the whole procedure, and think of a trigger word to remember when you're listening.*

A surreal shopping list?

I don't mind admitting that, having never been really ill, the prospect of regular hospital visits was filling me with dread, so to have something to distract my mind was very helpful.

35

A few run-throughs of the CD and I'm feeling somewhat less nervous, now it's off for the start of the hospital visits.

There could be rather a lot of these over the next few months.

The men in white coats.

I arrived, got out of the car and noticed I had sweaty palms.

'It's only a few scans, so calm down' I try telling myself, but my mind is full of *'what ifs?'*

Here goes.

First stop is back to St Anthony's in Cheam for an MRI scan. Into a back room. No natural light. I'm strapped down with a head, face and neck support. Just as well I'm not claustrophobic!

The medics leave the room. Just me and the scanner. The machine cranks up, decibel levels rising, and as I slide into the scan a metallic-sounding computerised voice issues the following instruction:

'Stop breathing'.

A minute or so later there has been no follow-up instruction which makes the whole thing seem even more surreal. It seems sensible to breathe again. The noise the machine makes is unbelievable!

All done in about an hour and it's off home. Tomorrow it's up to London for a PET/CT scan at some medical centre just off Harley Street. One more run-through of Suzi Smith's words of wisdom and I'm up for the next scan.

Starvation

My instructions before this next scan are: nothing to eat or drink for twelve hours previously, except very small amounts of water. Failure to adhere to the rules means no scan. All a little clinical and authoritarian in tone I can't help thinking.

I'd never considered a starvation diet would be the order of the day for scans, just one of many things I was going to learn.

I'd arrived at the clinically clean scan centre, had been escorted down to the basement, devoid of natural light, with everyone in white uniforms. I'd had to sign a few more forms and had been given a glass of water and a valium tablet to ensure I was 'relaxed' – not exactly my overriding feeling.

'This way Mr. Hern' as I'm led off to a small room, given a gown to wear, instructed to lie down, and left alone as the lights are dimmed. 'You'll be visited again in some twenty minutes, when you'll be injected with a glucose-based liquid to react with active cancer cells so they can be located on the scan,' I was advised before he disappeared and the door slammed shut behind him.

Silence.

This is all starting to feel a little like I'm part of some scientific experiment, or an extra in some sci-fi movie.

The nurse is back to inject the radioactive glucose, then it's lie still in near darkness for an hour before doing the scan. In another spotlessly clean, basement room.

'All staff leave the theatre and we'll switch him on' the order echoed around the theatre. This scan lasted only about forty minutes, was much quieter than the MRI, and scans the body in sections of a few inches at a time.

All done. Now the CT scan for close-up of the head and neck (the suspected location of the primary tumour) which requires an iodine injection.

'Don't worry if you feel some tightness in your neck, it'll be fine' says the nurse, in a practiced soothing voice, trying, but not succeeding, to make me feel at ease. It's fair to say what happened next scared the hell out of me – as the machine started up and I felt myself slowly sliding into the scanner, my neck started to contract. I just felt panic rising, visions of not being able to breathe, in spite of what I had been told. Fortunately it didn't last very long. *'Relax – they know what they are doing.'*

To me this is starting to feel like some kind of weird adventure, and I've only just begun whatever the hell the journey has in store. Scan complete I head for home with a parting warning from the medical centre staff ringing in my ears: 'don't go near any very young children, or pregnant women, for at least six hours as you will still be radio-active'.

I was left wondering just how strong this stuff is that they've just pumped me full of. It all seems so out of this world, but just then an amusing thought occurred to me.

'Does that mean I'll be like the Ready brek kid in the old 1970s TV ad, and glow as I walk down the street?'

Marital concern

This is day eight of 'living with cancer'. In some ways it already feels like far longer than that.

I get home, Madeleine's already there and is looking at a new book I have just started, 'Cosmic Ordering for Beginners'. One of the suggestions from the latest NLP session, this could not be described as an easy read, but it did further fuel my intrigue into the whole mental aspect.

Her face was an absolute picture, and she gave me what could best be described as an 'old-fashioned' look. I could almost hear her thinking *'what has happened to him – overdosed on radiation?'*

Strange what happens when a potentially life-ending issue disturbs your peaceful little world!

I reassure her the best I can that I'm still sane and not suffering from anything untoward!

Off for another game of golf, and no problems this week about the emotions. Even chat with the other guys about treatment and timescales. The only noticeable difference as far as they are concerned is my shorter than normal length of time in the 19th!

I left wondering how long I would be able to play for, but knowing I had an important responsibility to undertake.

Birthday

A house full of teenagers (Jess is 14 tomorrow) awaits. Instead of the fully fledged party this is a compromise due to my situation. A dozen or so friends, and I'm the chef on the barbecue. All goes really well, they're very….well, 'teenagerish'. Chat, chill, and play table football/pool, and then one wanders in to ask if I've got any old music. 'Like what?'

'Bon Jovi' comes the response. Putting on my best middle-aged-old-git expression I reply: 'that's not old. If you want old, I can do old. Rolling Stones, Pink Floyd, Bowie, Deep Purple, Black Sabbath….and so on….' In no time we were listening to The Stones at decibel levels I'm sure the neighbours enjoyed a lot. Followed in no time by Queen, and Led Zeppelin: have the 70s suddenly returned? I'm enjoying it and it's helping me forget the impending operation.

Jess' birthday itself was quite subdued by our standards. We did still manage to have the usual collection of street socialites round for the champagne and cake that is now tradition with any birthday. How lucky we are to live in such a great street, with such friendly, sociable neighbours.

As the last guest leaves I have that sinking feeling. The real stuff begins tomorrow. It's time for 'medical intervention' tomorrow, under the knife, and who knows what.

This is it then – the serious stuff starts now.

One more run-through of 'Preparing For A Medical Intervention', but this time I can't help feeling a bit edgy. Having never been in hospital other than to visit, the prospect of months of treatment is turning me into a bag of nerves.

Almost forgot. Quick dash to M&S to buy some pyjamas, not an item of clothing I've possessed since teenage years.

Now hospitalisation.......

3. Soup & Yoghurt

Medium-rare

Or at least that's how I felt, now half-way through the radiotherapy.

I imagine Helen anticipating my visit as the latest appointment time draws near. She is probably wondering what I'm looking like and how I'm coping.

I need this session to get the mental side back on track, as it has taken a bit of a kicking lately, and I've been feeling very low.

After listening carefully to my list of problems, she paused before suggesting I should view the whole treatment from a different angle. See it as a journey, every now and then a detour would be required (i.e. all those times when the treatment and its effects were getting me down), but remain focused on the destination and take the detours in my stride.

That's a very crude summary of over three hours hard work, but as usual I left in much better spirits and thinking more about '*only three weeks of treatment left*', and less on feeling so grim.

'*Funny how it goes – I'd never have considered working with a coach had it not been for the coincidental meeting with Helen.*'

'No such thing as coincidence' I can hear her saying. Whatever, I'm truly grateful for the help she has provided to help me to cope with the now numerous lows of the treatment.

I'm starting to notice the side effects of the treatment now. Lots of hair appearing on the bathroom floor whenever I have a shower was the first.

And no doubt connected to this is one of the weirder ones. At the beginning I was advised to get an electric shaver, as the usual wet shaving wouldn't work well with the radiotherapy being done on my neck.

What I hadn't realised was that this wouldn't be required for long. The radiotherapy soon stops any facial hair growth at all – indeed my neck and face were now feeling as soft as the proverbial baby's bottom. Very strange!

Probably the most consistent effect though is a persistent dry mouth, constantly needing to drink water.

Not being able to go more than a few minutes without a drink is a 24-hour-a-day situation now, so I've not had a proper night's sleep for a while, which just exacerbates the general lack of energy and overall tiredness.

As this has worsened so the benefit of a family driver to treatment has been enormous, another plus being Anna (my younger sister, and volunteer driver) is no slouch with the camera.

At the next weekly scan we start walking into the MRI room – 'don't bring the camera in here' shouts one of the nurses, 'it'll never work again!'

Maybe I can handle the radiation better than the camera.

I don the required uniform.

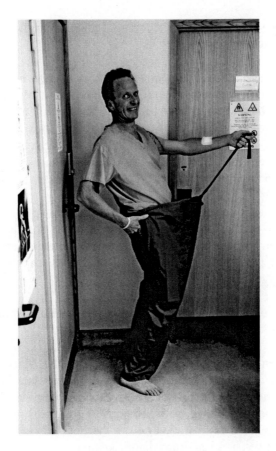

Hospital 'fashion'.

A brief escape

August bank holiday arrives and it's off to Glasgow for the weekend. Somehow it's not quite the same when the basic diet is soup and yoghurt, and all I can drink is water.

We stayed with an old friend and her new, slightly eccentric, boyfriend, before heading up to the coast, on to Glen Coe, and back round Loch Lomond. I've not been up here before, and the scenery is simply stunning. I must come back and do some photography.

I am struggling with a complete lack of energy, and severe boredom of soup and mineral water. Even so, it is nice to get away. There seem to have been trips lined up throughout the treatment, meaning I've always been able to look forward to the next one. I'm sure that has helped me through some of the darker times. The Really Big One is that massive holiday lined up for Christmas after everything is done and dusted.

Having an overseas trip to look forward to is, for me, an integral part of life generally. I'm always planning how, when and where to go next, along with the small matter of how to pay for it. Having visited over sixty countries, the next target is to top the hundred.

'Focus on the destination'. Helen's phrases do have a habit of popping up at opportune moments.

After an all-too-short break, it's back to the Marsden for another round of kidney tests prior to my last bout of chemotherapy – the results are depressingly familiar: kidney functionality is down, so I will need to go in early for a few extra hours of re-hydration before the hour of cisplatin (the first of two chemical drugs that make up my chemo).

I can only begin to imagine how strong this drug must be given the detailed tests required before it can be used. The consultant's initial few words echoed around my head 'do not underestimate just how hard your metabolism will be hit by the treatment – these are heavy duty chemical drugs'.

Last bout

So, back into the 'old room' and all those familiar faces on the nursing front – it's almost like coming home!

'How do they do it' I wonder. *Always cheerful, friendly, professional and caring, and in return for? Low pay, long hours, all in an environment full of sick people, some of whom don't survive'.* I know for sure I couldn't do it. How will I ever really be able to express my thanks and appreciation when I'm out?

Right now they have some further news for me. The latest batch of blood tests have shown up that there is something 'not quite right' with my white blood cells. I am assured this is a quite normal effect of the treatment, and easily rectified by a partial blood transfusion, so I'm hooked up to receive said transfusion. It's a little strange looking at someone else's blood being fed into my body. Strange but necessary I guess.

With a minimal appetite and not having been able to chew for weeks I have been shedding weight at a rapid rate, and during this, my last stay in hospital, I am despatched to the dietician. One of the folk that want to fill me full of tubes and force-feed me.

'God I don't want that. How can it be avoided?'

The dietician is very keen on going down the route of force-feeding, something that's not a quick procedure. Apparently I would need the tube in for months if this is the route taken.

Got a check-up with Andrew Jones coming up – see what he thinks.

'Oh yes, they are always keen on force-feeding, but it's not necessary yet.'

'Yet?' I ask hesitantly.

'You must start eating more to avoid it.'

So easy to say. I can't chew, can't taste anything, trying to eat has gradually become a real chore.

Fortunately, I am in the capable hands of two constant 'bullies' in the form of two nurses, Claire and Kim. Chatty, cheerful and with great senses of humour.

'Listen... ' I am instructed.

New food ideas

'Try such things as 'sinking' a piece of bread into the bowl of soup, and start eating sweet biscuits that can be dunked in tea. Anything that increases the calorie count, but doesn't require chewing.'

Now the last chemo top-up, and I'm not looking forward to this, as the last one made me feel so dire. Need to take some pre-chemo precautions – this time more and stronger anti-vomit medication are both provided.

Try to look on the bright side – it's the last chemo session!

Done, and the extra dosage has really helped.

I am also loaded up with dietary supplements ranging from milk shakes, to specially formulated fruit drinks, to Calogen which is basically liquid fat. Sounds vile!

The peak of medication has now been reached and my daily intake is a rather impressive:

Anti-vomit/painkillers:
- Dexamothasone steroids two tablets, three times a day
- Granisitron anti-vomit, one daily
- Metoclopramide anti-vomit, three times a day
- Dissolved aspirin, three times a day

Other medication:

- Tyler effervescent, two tablets three times a day
- Chlorhexide Gluconote (mouthwash in English), four times a day
- Radiance skin cream , three-four times daily
- Gelkam tooth gel, twice daily

Food supplements – as much of these as can be achieved:

Two milk shake additions
Two spoons of Calogen with each meal
As much of the fruit drink as possible

'Oh, and could you try to get some food down, as well as all this lot?'

'Leave it with me, I'll see what I can do!' The 'quiet motivator', Kim, stops by for a chat when I'm preparing to leave my second home, with one of 'her expressions'. *'What's she going to come up with?'* She's a real character never short of a comment or two.

'So what do you get up to when you're not lounging around occupying one of our much-needed hospital beds?' she says with a wry smile.

'I'm a freelance photographer'. I replied.

'Oh great', says she 'I need you'.

'Best offer I've had in ages'.

'No, seriously, I'm getting married next year – would you do the wedding photography?'

'Of course I will – it would be a pleasure, even though you've done not a lot for me. Except maybe help me live'.

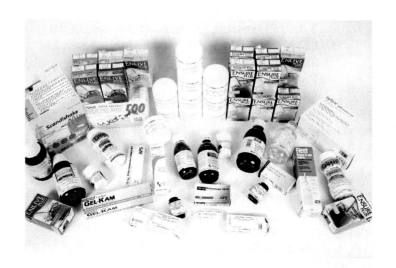

'Complete' medication.

Final round

I feel really tired and weak after this last bout of chemotherapy.

'Nearly done. Hang on in there. You can do it.'

My food and drink intake has shrunk enormously, and even with these supplements and is way below the required daily calorie intake. By means of example this is all I could manage for two days on the 4th and 5th September:

4th September:

Breakfast:

Bowl of Rice Crispies, milk, sugar	white coffee
	Scandishake
	500ml water

Lunch:

Two mouthfuls of mushed steak pie	250g Maxidual
Tomato & crème fraiche soup	250ml water
1 piece of white bread (sunk in the soup)	

Dinner:

Bowl of four bean & lentil soup	500ml water
Raspberry jelly, custard, double cream	1 cup Lucozade

5th September:

Breakfast:

Rice Crispies, milk, sugar	white coffee
Poached egg	500ml water

Lunch:

Fried egg, tinned tomatoes	flat Coca Cola 500ml
Chopped tinned pears, custard, double cream	250g Maxidual
Dunked shortbread biscuit	white tea

Dinner:

Tomato build-up soup, sunken bread Chopped tinned pears, custard	500ml water

Anyway, quickly back into the familiar routine of the daily radiotherapy. My new mate Mel is now suffering. She's having a really tough time with her mouth full of ulcers so eating is painful, and has also reached dry-throat stage so can't chew.

My turn to start cheering her up, or at least I hope I can. Discussions focus on when we've both got our tastes back. It's agreed, we'll meet up for an extremely over-indulgent lunch when conditions allow.

The daily queue for radiotherapy is a long way from a cheerful environment. Ten to twenty minutes in a line of glum faces, most very pale. Grim!

I ponder *'how much harder would this last bit have been without Mel's ready wit and repartee?'*

The end of the treatment is fast approaching now, but I've suddenly been hit with a new side-effect. Weeks of no solids, no energy, no full night's sleep, and now: I can't even perform the basic of basic functions, and find myself constipated to an unbelievably painful extent.

'What else is going to happen? How much more discomfort will I have to suffer? This is so painful......

Yet more medication required to get rid of yet another unwelcome side effect. More pills and even suppositories. Tears well up in my eyes. It just feels like my private humiliation is complete, like my whole body is just packing up, to go with the hair loss, weight loss, inability to eat or chew, no proper sleep, no energy, always tired.

I feel like I'm in physical meltdown. At this late stage of treatment is it finally going to grind me into submission and beat me? Is this it?

'Think of it as a journey, you are on one of those detours', a soft, re-assuring voice appears somewhere in my head *'hang on in there, almost over'.*

It's check-up time again.

I bring moral support, and Mads joins me for my next session with Andrew Jones. He's very pleased with how the treatment is going – he beckons her over to look inside my mouth, graphically explains how it looks like a strawberry in the front half, and the back half is full of this yellowy phlegm.

Where is that camera when it's needed?

Radiotherapy finishes

The 13th September arrives and my last radiotherapy session is here – a date I shall never forget. On the one hand I'm relieved to see the back of this, and on the other depressed that there is still, what did they say?, a couple of weeks more of going downhill.

Say cheerio to my Mel, re-confirm we will arrange that drunken lunch, say thanks to the radiotherapy team and I'm a free man again.

My neck has survived amazingly well – thanks totally to the Radiance cream from the Bristol (Penny Brohn) Cancer Centre that I've been using. At £16 a tub it's not cheap, but having seen my neighbour's neck during my first bout of chemo treatment, I felt every one of the nine tubs I got through was worth the expense! Strangely the medics weren't overly impressed with my choice of skin-cream – never did understand why, when it worked so well for me.

How long until I start seeing some improvement?

Back to life

First social event was an invitation to Stamford Bridge to watch a Chelsea match. (I've been a supporter, mainly of the armchair type, since watching them lose to Spurs in the 1967 Cup Final). A special invitation as I managed to get an invite to the press box as a 'regular journo'.

I arrived in time for the delicious-looking roast lamb with all the trimmings, and an impressive array of desserts and cheeses. This is a bit different to the usual hot dog on the terraces (it's a while since I've been to a game!).

'Thanks, but just a soup and glass of water for me!' *'This diet is so dull, I wonder if I'll ever look at another bowl of soup after the taste returns? I need to work on an invite back here to sample this haute cuisine when I can eat again.'*

Two important dates stand out. The 21st September has been in the diary since pre-cancer as the targeted first date for any kind of gentle exercise – a day's golf.

The second and vital target is the end of October. Plenty of determined training required to make this a success. We are off for a weekend to Tuscany. Plenty of eating meats, game, cheese, pasta and maybe the odd glass or two of the local wine. Six weeks to get to the stage where I can chew a meal, and even drink wine, let alone taste it. Given the current state of affairs that won't be easy, but seems like a good target!

Plus a local photo exhibition to arrange at the end of September with a private view evening, to which between fifty and a hundred people will be coming.

To keep my sanity through the darker times, of which there have been plenty, and apart from the obvious benefit of Helen's work, I have found it vital to have targets to aim for outside the treatment.

Anything from small ones like a game of golf, to the much larger ones, which tend to be overseas trips. It doesn't really matter what, just something positive to think about. It's really helped break up the monotony of the treatment, the diet, feeling awful, having no energy and so on.

Strong family support back home certainly helps, although God knows what Mads and Jess have been through the last few months. What towers of strength they have been.

A phrase suddenly springs to mind '*You find out who your real friends are when you need them most*'. It's certainly thrown up a few surprises, or perhaps it's just that everyone has their own way of handling the situation.

First round

The 21st September is here, and I make it up to Swinley Forest for the golf event – I can only do one round, need a buggy, and can't handle lunch. Chat with the guys about where I am with treatment, particularly one who went through cancer himself a couple of years ago. There seem an awful lot of people who've been through this, or is it just I notice it more nowadays?

A really enjoyable morning, finished playing not too badly, which always helps, before it's off home. The excitement's been too much and I need to lie down! That is the most energetic I have been for a couple of months or so.

The next day we'd been invited down to a friend's house-warming. A new house, and the start of a new life after separating from his wife. I have to bring my own refreshments – yet more soup and mineral water, none of that tasty looking Italian spread and decent wine. *If only!*

'When, when, when will I get my taste back?'

Dietary supplements

Although the treatment is now over the side effects are still increasing. The desire for food is not getting any better, the weight loss is now over two stone and I didn't carry much in the way of excess anyway.

No choice but to start trying these dietary supplements provided by the hospital as the risk of being force-fed through a tube is still here.

'Let's start with these fortified fruit drinks'. My taste buds may be shot to bits but these are awful – will have to try again, but 'yuk'! Next, the milk-shake supplements – just

about manageable, but only to the tune of one a day as far as I was concerned. I was supposed to have two.

'Now for the 'liquid fat' – sounds great! The real calorie intake, Calogen, was something else. I managed a few spoonfuls to start with, but liquid fat isn't exactly appealing. Persevering, it was about the third attempt when I managed a spoonful, and instantly threw up: thick, bright orange liquid all over the place! Next time stay near the sink.

I approached the next attempt with due trepidation. Try the strawberry one this time. It's down. For all of ten seconds before I vomit it all up, and the sink is covered in pink mess. That's it, I can't do this, the end of this dietary supplement experiment.

Surreal

Treatment finished days ago, side-effects are worsening, and it's still weeks until I can go through all the tests and scans again to see if it's worked. Something of a 'surreal phase'. My head is struggling to cope with this – the treatment ended seemingly ages ago, and I'm just deteriorating.

I've now lost so much weight I can feel bones poking through in areas I never knew I had them! When diagnosed I weighed in at around 13 stone and 4 pounds, but now I'm fighting not to fall much below 11 stone. I have lost most of the hair on the back of my head, I don't have any clothes that fit any more but, most importantly....

'I'm still here!

'Surely it can't be too much longer before something happens. Remember many who get this disease don't make it! I know, but now I'm just impatient for some sign, no matter how small'.

The havoc cancer has been playing with my brain is still here. One minute trying to be positive that the end of treatment is close, the next a sea of depression as nothing seems to get better.

4. Chemicals & Chemo

Chemotherapy

Back to the early stage of treatment, and the hospital visit immediately pre-chemo. I was informed that this consisted of a 'morning of tests on kidney functionality' (EDTA to get technical), basically to check they will withstand the chemical attack that's about to take place.

I make it into the Marsden well before the appointed 9.15, and am eventually seen at about 9.50. Maybe the medical world operates on a different time zone. I guess it's pretty difficult to predict accurately how long each patient appointment is going to take. The technician explains he'll take a blood test first then fill me full of some other chemical (at this rate I'll have ticked off the whole of the periodic elements table, or whatever it was called).

Then I'm dispatched and told to come back in three hours to take another blood test. I'm starting to feel a little like a pin-cushion. They will then test how much of the said chemical the kidneys have processed, which tells how effectively they are working.

So, my 'morning of tests' turns out to be two five minute visits and three hours wandering around central London.

My last evening of freedom, and with hospital looming there is time for one last takeaway curry. I just make sure I enjoy the chicken madras, pilau rice, tarka dall, brinjal bhaji and nan bread. *'When will the next one be?'* Same old thought pattern again.

'Chemo day' arrives and, perhaps unsurprisingly, I'm feeling somewhat less relaxed this morning. A feeling not helped when our front drain blocks and leaves the place smelling like a sewage farm. Not an ideal start, but certainly keeps the mind off the treatment (I can almost hear Helen *'no such thing as a coincidence'*).

Arrange for the drain clearers to turn up, then focus on something really important. Getting enough tunes onto the iPod for what could be quite a lot of listening over the next few days. A neighbour has popped by with some music to lend me, laughingly dismissing my iPod 'shuffle' as being woefully inadequate for the job in hand, and insisting I use his. He deletes all of his tunes and copies my selection – fantastic.

This done, drain cleared, it's time to go, and Mads and I head off.

Check-in

'I've come to check in to your smart hotel' say I to the guy on the reception.

'That's fine, Mr?'

'Hern.'

'Unfortunately the room with the sea view is gone.'

'Sorry not good enough, I'd like to see the manager'.

'Another bloody comedian' I can almost hear him say, but as ever a little laugh here and there really helps. Off for some more blood tests (the results of the kidney tests yesterday were fine). Little did I know at this stage just how many times over the forthcoming months I would have a blood test.

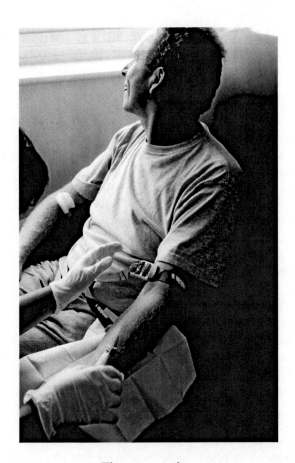

The new routine.

I was met by Anne, the admissions lady, who took on what felt like a complete tour of the hospital. Suffice to say I had no idea where we ended up, except it was on the top floor. She put a cannula (the link into the vein through which the chemo is dispensed) in my arm, took me to the Weston ward, and the funny little room down the corridor, and round the corner, where I am staying.

It's even equipped with a closed circuit TV camera pointed at the bed. Shane, a jovial Australian nurse, helpfully pointed out 'it's so far for the nurses to walk that it's more efficient to keep an eye on you through the TV, and don't worry because we'll come out the moment we seeing you lying on the floor in a pool of blood'.

'I'll sleep better knowing that!'

By now it's a couple of hours or so after arriving and it doesn't look like I'll be hooked up (or should that be tuned in? switched on?) until later in the evening as all the chemo bits are in the lab and the concoction is being created.

'Bubble, bubble toil and trouble' has nothing on this.

Procession of 'medics'

Mads is with me and watches with wry amusement at the sheer number of staff that drop by to say hi, and the immense number of forms required that Aussie Shane goes through. He's a contract nurse, who works hospitals here in the summer and goes to Austria for the winter – seems to have more appeal than a cancer ward if you ask me.

Next a doctor appears and calmly states she going to give me a quick examination – sensing my nervousness she smiles and explains helpfully 'don't worry it's just like an MOT on a car'.

'Will my body of early Morris Minor vintage manage this?' I wonder.

No problem. Sailed through the MOT. '58 must have been a good vintage! She then moves onto those lifestyle questions to which I know she will be, how can I say it, 'underwhelmed' with my answers.

'Do you smoke and drink?' (I stopped smoking over nine years ago, and yes drink more than medically advised, maybe fifty units a week).

Is that 'one five or five zero' says she? 'Five zero' I reply.

The stony silence that followed made me feel like a school kid who was just about to be given a detention. Tutting disapprovingly at my answer she asked 'when was the last time you went five days without a drink, as you can't have any in here?' 'Er, not sure, a while ago!' To which she suggested I might suffer withdrawal symptoms so they'd be watching me for that as well. Dr. Disapproving?

'Oh great, as if having cancer's not bad enough.'

Another nurse appeared seemingly only to re-emphasise what the likely common side effects of the chemo would be, and left me with 'some' more detail. The list is nothing short of impressive. For the cisplatin/ 5-fluoro-uracil chemo treatment (my 'carefully chosen' chemical mix) they are:

      tiredness
      loss of appetite
      altered taste
      indigestion
      diarrhoea or constipation
      mouth ulcers
      vomiting
      altered hearing
      neuropathy
      infections and blood clots
      possible hair loss
      not to mention infertility
      the long shot of a fatal complication related to blood clots
      the possibility of needing a blood transfusion

'Is that all? Should be a breeze then', I joke, although feeling anything but humorous at that list. In reality I feel ill just at the thought.

After another load of paperwork she continues, 'once you've handled this little lot and the chemotherapy is complete, then it's a break and into radiotherapy', which by all popular accounts is the part of the treatment during which I will feel worst, or at least that's what the consultants made sure I was fully aware of.

The radiotherapy side effect list includes:

>skin breakdown
>inability to chew
>pain and discomfort when swallowing and eating which may even become impossible, and if so then a tube is fed either up your nose and down your throat, or just straight into the stomach (can hardly wait!)
>sore mouth
>loss of taste
>altered voice (try not to talk much on radiotherapy was the useful advice)
>hair loss on the back of the head
>tiredness
>persistently dry mouth

Well, what a fun-packed few weeks I have coming up. As there's no choice anyway, better get started on the premise that the sooner it's started, the sooner it's finished.

Any pretence I had about being relaxed has completely gone now to be replaced by a level of trepidation I am unfamiliar with.

Naked fear would be a more accurate way of putting it, and a more realistic assessment of my current mental state.

Hook-up time

Having now met, seemingly, the entire medical staff of the Marsden, during which time I also seemed to have signed my life away on numerous bits of documentation in my first few hours. Some are explanatory, many to avoid risk of litigation in case something untoward should happen. Legal action never seems far from any area of life these days. *'I can't remember ever coming across a poor lawyer'*.

Anna, my younger sister, was the first visitor, so just bought her up to speed before she produced a couple of packs of cards for a quick game of Canasta. It's been so long I had completely forgotten she plays by a totally different set of rules, with the predictable consequence – I get soundly thrashed!

The time has finally arrived. With all the reliability of a railway timetable the afternoon start is about ten o'clock at night when the first drip is put in. This is just a saline solution to flush my system through, and the nurse will be back in four hours to swap this for a few more short drips, before getting the main line (for the chemo compound 5FU) in by about three or four in the morning, so have a good sleep!

I wonder how many tests, how many trials, and how many patients that don't make it has it taken to know for sure this is the right concoction of drugs, in the right mix, to be administered over the right length of time, with the right number of breaks in the treatment...... the mind boggles!

Drop off to sleep, but awoken by a sound that will become very familiar over the next few days, 'the beeping drip'. Wearily I look at my watch - it's about 2 a.m. and the drip's empty. The nurse arrives, and attaches the next drip which is thirty minutes of an anti-sickness drug, then an hour of the first chemo drug cisplatin.

I had been told this is *'the'* really heavy-duty chemo chemical. It looks just the same as the 'flush through' to the naked eye – appearances can be deceptive!

It's a little creepy watching this clear solution being fed into my system, about which my total knowledge is nothing more than it's 'heavy duty'. Then another thirty minute flush-through, and finally the 5FU is linked up at around 3.30.... I'm shattered.

I awake around seven and now need to acquire a new skill – moving around whilst attached to a drip. Normal movement is impossible, so having a shower/bath needs the drip properly taken out; strange what little things normally taken for granted need someone else to assist, but all the nurses so far encountered are so good and kind it's not a problem.

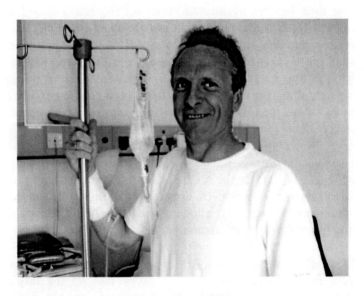

Chemotherapy starts.

Breakfast (shades of school dinners), a room clean, blood pressure & pulse tests all done, I'm ready for the arrival of 'the gang'. Something of a ritual for us new arrivals. A squad of consultants, senior doctors, junior doctors et al, about eight in all, come to inspect the latest admission. It's bit like being the new arrival in a zoo.

All seems okay, and they ask if I would mind being involved in a couple of clinical trials – someone will drop by explain more the nurse nonchalantly tells me.

'We'll send another doctor in later to go through these in more detail, so you can sign up for them'. Next up my other sister, Jane, arrives – she's come all the way up from deepest Sussex just to have a chat for an hour or so. How sweet of her!

Then Mads arrives – great that her work are being so understanding - and really nice to see her.

'So what have you been up to then?' she asks

'Pull up a chair, this might take a while!'

The tooth lady!

I've been advised I need to see the resident dentist, so am taken down to the depths of the hospital to check if my teeth are in good enough condition for the treatment, for a full dental x-ray and check-up. Until now it hadn't occurred to me that my teeth might be involved, but with my dental history that was unlikely to bring good news.

There was quite a queue so I got talking with another patient who'd been diagnosed with a similar cancer to me, and he was just about to have two wisdom teeth pulled, so his four day sailing holiday starting tomorrow was about to become history.

He was not in a good way – edgy, upset, tearful. It turned out he was a hypnotherapist who dealt in phobias/fears affecting others – this was different, very real and affecting him, and it showed.

Having obviously read some of the information about the 'fertility issues of the treatment' he had come straight here from the sperm bank as he and his wife hadn't started a family, but with the strong chance of being infertile he wanted to cover all possibilities. If he managed to 'produce' under this level of stress I take my hat off to the man – good on him!

Onward to the dentist, 'Miss Holmes'. *Don't these medics have Christian names?*

She had a quick look round my mouth, said I'd need two (possibly three) teeth out, and would need to get some special fluoride. This I'd need to rub onto all of my teeth and gums morning and night for a week before radiotherapy, all the way through radio, and then once a day for ever after that.

'What if I don't?'

'You'll get a nasty infection which will turn all your teeth black and rotten!'

'In that case, OK!'

With radiotherapy and poor teeth (which I have in spades), not mixing, I casually ask if it wouldn't be better to replace them all and save me loads of dental bills in the future? She smiled, and replied that if we were in the US that is exactly what would happen.

I asked about this clinical trial I've agreed to do (modified lasering angles for the radiotherapy to minimise damage to the glands that produce saliva as dry mouth syndrome is very common after radiotherapy).

She replied 'that's fine for the glands themselves, but the long, wiggly bits' – I looked at her quizzically, both of us dissolving into laughter, as did the other two assistants, when she realised what she had just said.

'The what?' asked I, after the laughter had subsided.

'That'll be what joins the glands to the mouth - the ducts'.

'I think long, wiggly bits sounds far better!'

The characters

With the dental check-up duly completed it's back up to the room to find that new medication has appeared. Some clinical mouthwash I have to gargle with four times a day and different sickness prevention pills. The number of pills I have to take is rising steadily now. I have just started on a steroid called Dexamethasone three times a day for three days, plus the anti-sickness Metoclopramide also three times a day for three days.

'I thought hospital was supposed to be deadly boring, rather than the current steady stream of visitors' I pondered as the next arrived. Dr Alexander is here to go through another clinical trial I've been asked to consider.

At present they use the results of the CAT scan for locating the tumour and the precise focusing of the laser treatment, but have a belief that the MRI scan could provide more precise detail, thus allowing even more focused radiotherapy. Sounds like a good idea to me.

'So can you use the results to further fine-tune my treatment?' I asked. 'No, it's too early in the trial', but as all that is entailed for me is to go for another MRI scan I said that would be fine. She left me with all the documentation to approve. I've completely lost count of the number of bits of paper I've signed so far!

This place is full of characters, and that's just the staff. There's the 'red team leader', a delightful lady by the name of Claire who is very much into her holidays, and had just come back from Croatia, having already been to Egypt, and the South of France (which apparently didn't count as she stayed at a relatives!), and had also done Australia, Malaysia and Thailand. Excellent news as that should provide plenty of scope for travel-chat, a favourite topic of mine.

Then there's the night nurse from Cape Town who used to work at Robben Island before the end of apartheid, when Nelson Mandela was prisoner. She had never met the man himself, but I'm sure she's got some fascinating stories! She and her husband, who is also in the medical world over here, only manage to get back to South Africa every other year, due mainly to the rip-off air fares prevalent over Christmas. This is the only time of year they can both get the time off. Don't I know that problem as Christmas is our favourite time of year to be somewhere hot.

Next there's the Irish day nurse, Maggie, with that wonderful accent and laid-back style of the Irish. I used to go over to Ireland regularly for golf weekends in pre-parenthood days, and Maggie seemed to know all the best courses. The subject soon turned to Guinness and the inevitable 'you can't get proper Guinness anywhere except Ireland'. Apparently her father refuses to drink the stuff anywhere but Ireland.

The mobile 'text alert' message rings out – *'Dad, can I come up and stay on Friday night?'* Permission given, great!

Jess is being really strong over my situation, but I know it's affecting her, particularly this week as I'm in hospital. She has one of the leading roles in the school drama production of 'Grease' in which she has two solos – she has a great voice these days, and will be fine. A girl's father is, of course, always the most reliable source for a truly unbiased assessment of her abilities!

One last visit from Sue to check I'm still here, and then it's off to sleep until the 3.30 alarm call for the change of 5FU drips. Uncanny how it always happens in the middle of the night. More to the point, Sue has sneaked off and found a substitute to swap my drip tonight!

Waking up around 6.30 and it's the now usual morning routine: blood pressure, pulse and weigh-in. Thought I might try the next Suzi Smith CD – 'Creating a Healthy Identity'. This, I'm afraid proved all too much, and went completely over my head!

It seems odd that I'm busy reading all this stuff, but I'm finding it really helpful in terms of keeping my mind on the positive.

Now fully conversant (small exaggeration) with the world of 'Cosmic Ordering' next up on the wacky reading list is 'The Secret', which apparently has attracted a fair amount of publicity so will have to see what that's all about.

Work?

The mobile rang and it was one of my largest customers (he of the Camberwell pub shoot), but it had been a few weeks since we'd spoken.

'Hi Keith, what are the chances you could do a photo shoot for me this evening in Piccadilly Circus?'

'Could be tricky –I'm in hospital'.

'What time will you be available then?'

'No, I'm not visiting, it's me that's in for treatment'.

After somewhat of a pause, 'nothing serious I hope?'

There's a question. 'Bit early to tell, except to say it's cancer, but they know how to treat it'.

'Good luck'. He says, not quite sure how to react.

'Thanks, I'll be in touch when I'm back in the normal world'.

He is the first of my business contacts to hear of my condition, but I assure him I will be back in touch as soon as I'm out.

Mads arrives later the morning with the all-important timesonline article, which was really well placed in the paper. Next time I must remember to run spell check on an article before submitting anything as there are not one, but three, glaring typos, and, yes, all in the first few lines.

Yet more medical visitors. First off is Mr Cheadle to go through the clinical trial for the throat, so duly signed yet more paperwork for this. Hopefully this will help save at least some of the saliva-producing glands to survive the forthcoming onslaught.

Then a speedy visit from Doctor Disapproving (she who had put me on 'withdrawal symptom' watch) and the subject of the radiotherapy cropped up. Another re-statement of how uncomfortable this is likely to be, and how some patients need tubes to feed from, and can forget how to swallow. All in all a really cheery summary!

They don't hold back when explaining the 'delights' of what the treatment is likely to do. Her last instruction was, between now and the radiotherapy, to 'eat, eat and eat, and eat again, as much as you can, and make it as calorie-rich as possible – you'll need it later'.

God she made it sound even more dreadful – quick change subjects.

'So what will I be able to do next week when I'm home?' I enquire.

'Lead a normal life, but be very aware of what your body is telling you' she replied. *'That's a bit cryptic'.*

Last, but most certainly not least, 'will I be okay to go to Italy on July 20th?' I ask somewhat nervously.

'Should be fine'.

Result! Instantly I'm in a much better mood – it's always the same whenever an overseas trip is booked.

I decide it's time to go and meet my next door neighbour, who seemed to be having a tough time. Her neck looked like it had second degree burns, she can't eat, is having trouble speaking, and is generally struggling.

So this was what radiotherapy was going to be like.

My early evening check-up visit from Sue duly arrived (it turns out she's Anne's mum, the admissions lady that met me on arrival on Tuesday). Conversation drifted onto the 'C' word, and she admitted to shedding a tear or two when one of her favourite patients was told nothing more could be done, and he duly passed away (he was John Diamond who wrote a book while in here 'Cowards Get Cancer Too').

An involuntary shiver went down my spine - I've never experienced being in a situation where death is a regular occurrence, and very much part of daily routine. I'm tempted to ask what proportion of patients leave the hospital in a pine box, but decide not to as I might not like the answer.

If I thought I was feeling confident previously, this was a reality wake up call – *'I may not get through this.'*

'Just how do the nurses do this day in and day out, with death being such a common part of life?' – how can they seemingly switch off when they leave for home? They must, as otherwise they'd crack up. So many questions....'

I must admit to being in awe of what a fantastic job they do, and, from my limited experience in such good spirits!

Radio chat

While not feeling too bad, I thought I'd ask Sue just how grim radiotherapy is likely to be, just to see if her prognosis was as dire as the others. It was. She recounted how difficult it is likely to be to swallow, eat, taste, talk and explained in graphic detail how if a feeding tube is required, some are put through the nose and down the throat, others straight into the stomach – nice choice!

'Just make sure you eat as much as possible between now and when radiotherapy starts, particularly high calorie foods - you'll need it'. After imparting this piece of advice she turns and leaves, and I feel my mindset taking a rapid turn for the worse.

After a mixed night's sleep I awake thinking about the patient next door – it sounded like she had just had a really bad night with coughing up that thick mucus every couple of hours. I dropped round a while later, and she did seem in brighter spirits, but those noises on top of all the news yesterday about radiotherapy had left me feeling very low and slightly tearful this morning. Needing to get the mind occupied again I reached for Lance Armstrong's book 'It's Not About The Bike' and started reading.

I was getting rapidly ensconced in Lance's experiences when the message alert went on the mobile. The numerous 'don't use a mobile in hospital as it could interfere with medical equipment' warnings always did sound rather suspect to me.

Was it a coincidence that they were always trying to persuade you to use the hospital phones? Judging by the cost I have a slight suspicion it's more to do with making money, or perhaps meeting another set of meaningless 'government targets'.

The message was from Glenn Edwards (award winning Welsh photographer, and all-round great guy, who led the Gambian photo trip I went on in spring 2005) who, apart from specialising in interesting conversations with various authorities of central African countries, wanted a chat about starting up a photo library based on travel. Sounds good to me.

In no time at all I had another visitor. I should have opened a 'guest book' when I first came in here. Caroline, from the speech and language therapy unit, had dropped in to discuss tongue exercises in preparation for the side-effects of radiotherapy.

'Are you serious?' I asked.

'Absolutely, this will ensure that you will be able to keep the correct movement in your tongue as you go through radiotherapy', she said in all seriousness. The advice entitled 'Tongue Exercises: the aim is to increase the movement and strength of the tongue', goes as follows:

1. stick your tongue out, with your mouth wide open. Hold for one second then release.
2. lift your tongue up in your mouth. Hold for one second then release.
3. stick your tongue out to the right. Hold for one second then release. Now do the same to the left.
4. hold tongue firmly between the front teeth or gums and swallow.
5. pull your tongue back in your mouth. Hold for one second then release.
6. imagine gargling.

7. using a wettened spatula stick your tongue out and push against the left side of your tongue. Hold for one second and repeat to the right.

Repeat 1-7 times. Repeat entire set five times a day.

After a few minutes training I was now fully equipped with these tongue movements – now where are those 'gurning championships?'

Radiotherapy just seems like a never-ending list of problems. I will need to keep working on the mental side to get through this. A few words from Lance Armstrong's *'It's not About the Bike'* came to mind. 'Why not make the impossible possible?' was what he decided after being given minimal chance of survival – he went on to achieve the impossible.

The power of a positive thought! It worked for him.

'Taste'

Jess is coming up to stay tonight and I can't wait. She's even selected what video we'll be watching so it should be fun.

I suddenly notice that my wallet has gone walk-about. It had been in the bedside cabinet under some magazines, and even so some little scumbag has nicked it. Unbelievably, it's obviously commonplace, as I now notice all the warning signs in the wards and the corridors.

Stealing from cancer patients hooked up on chemotherapy – how low is that?

Mads turns up with Jess and I'm just ecstatic to see her. She's come with a huge get well soon card that she's got a load of school-mates and friends in the street to sign. I can't hold it together and let a few tears roll down the cheeks.

These raised level of emotions, I am informed, are apparently another (yet another?) common side-effect of the treatment.

How many more are there? I wonder.

Mads doesn't stay for too long as I suspect she's looking forward to catching up on some well-earned sleep: she's been incredibly strong, but even she must be feeling the strain of the last month. Anyway, Jess has already selected the movie, and produced the goodies that she collected at 'Taste' the previous evening.

'Taste' seems a somewhat apt name for an event I missed out on due to the current circumstances, but it's basically an evening strolling around Regent's Park sampling food and drink from the top chefs and best restaurants in London. How ironic. I am left thinking '*will I be okay come next year's event?*'

Just before the movie I show off my array of tongue-strengthening exercises, which unsurprisingly has Jess in near hysterics.

'Come on Jess, this is serious stuff ...' can't even finish the sentence before we're laughing again.

It's so good having her up to stay.

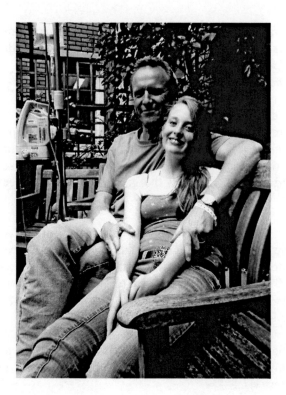

Cheering up the old man.

That's for another day. Now we settle down on the bed to watch 'Hot Fuzz', her ladyship's choice of movie. It's just a delight to be with her and both dozing off in front of a movie.

That familiar bleeping at 3.30 so wake up for a change of drip. I'm sure the timing is deliberate, but at least it's the last one. On the home stretch of part one, but strangely can't get back to sleep for a couple of hours. Jess stirs around 7.30 and reckoned the fold-down was probably the least comfortable bed she has ever encountered. Anyway, up and showered she disappeared out of the hospital to go and find her own breakfast somewhere in SW7... as any self-respecting fourteen year old would do!

The 'neighbour' drops by. She's been in for six days, has another two weeks to go and is well into her radiography and the side-effects.

She hasn't managed to eat for nine days, and doesn't even feel like it! As a result they will be fitting that auto-feed tube straight into the stomach. In conjunction with the noises emanating from her room at night it doesn't sound good. She's virtually lost her voice, but after a few minutes I can just about understand her, and swap the mutual 'we'll be okay, we'll get through this', although looking at her state I'm not so sure.

Home tomorrow – and it can't come a minute too soon.

Back home

3.30 a.m. and the chemo's over. I'm detached from the drip and no more 5FU or cisplatin for sixteen days. What a relief that is – round one complete!

Mads appears bang on eight o'clock, and all of a sudden I feel really emotional. Can't explain it, feels very odd, but nearly in tears at the prospect of going home. The realisation I'm still here? A side-effect of six days on chemicals? or what? Don't understand this – very weird.

Anyway, arrive at home and greeted by a big hug from Jess – that always feels great, even more so now. Needless to say I've come home with all kinds of 'medical goodies' starting with a card I need to have with me at all times.

'This patient is on Cytotoxic Chemotherapy'. *'Should that be preceded by a large red warning sign 'Keep Clear?'*

I am under strict instructions to contact the hospital immediately if I feel any one of eight effects.

As well as this I'm armed with more mouthwash, anti-vomit pills to be taken three times a day for the next seven days, plus two tubes of 'tooth-rub' to avoid the dental issues surrounding the effects of radiotherapy. The walking pharmacy is here, and fine.

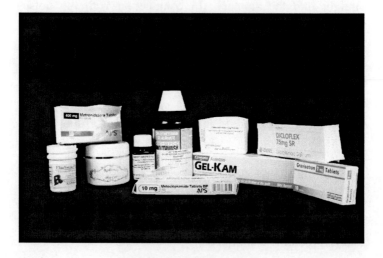

Early stage medication.

As the evening arrives and my first day back at home comes towards its close I feel a strange mixture of emotions. Absolutely ecstatic at getting through the first week with no major issues, and particularly pleased that the chemo seems to have sorted out the secondary tumour already (or at least shrunk it to the point of not being able to feel it).

On the other hand, this morning's strange emotional blip caught me out completely, the radiotherapy is getting closer and after what I've seen and heard in the last five days I need further work on the mental front.

I wake as though I was expecting the drip to be changed i.e. about 4 a.m., and for some reason don't really sleep properly afterwards. Mads has slept in another room to try to avoid passing on her cold – shame as it would have been really nice to snuggle up close to her after five nights apart.

How strong?

Mads leaves for work, departing with a cautionary 'take it easy, remember what the hospital said about over-doing it, and just relax!' A farewell kiss, and, 'of course not darling'.

Thought I'd just run the vacuum around a couple of rooms downstairs. Twenty minutes later and I'm flat out, knackered on the settee, and sleep solidly for two hours.

'*Just how strong are these chemo chemical concoctions I've spent six days having pumped into me?*'

After that little experience I opt for the less energetic approach, and lounge around not doing much (read a bit, listened to some Suzi Smith – still can't get my head around 'Communicating With Your Symptoms') until my parents turned up around 11.30. They were obviously highly relieved to see that I still look pretty much the same, and handed me a parcel that had been left on the doorstep.

An Amazon package - I hadn't ordered anything, so opened it with intrigue – it was a present of a photo book from some of Madeleine's work mates. The tears rolled again. That's two strange emotional outbursts in just over 24 hours – very odd, but apparently not totally unusual: just the chemo? Another mental affect of the 'c' word? who knows?

Either way it's another unexpected example of kindness. I am starting to find this somewhat of a humbling experience. Something deep inside tells me I'll come through this a better person. Don't know how or why, but it's just a feeling. Another little something else that I can't begin to explain.

Calories and more calories.....

'*Get a grip*', I tell myself. I can see the surprise on Mum's face at my reaction. 'Don't worry it's the drugs', I advise her, unconvincingly.

Off to The Swan, our riverside local, for some serious calorific intake, as instructed.

How ironic that I've only recently come off a course of statin pills to bring down my cholesterol, and now I'm straight back on 'the lard-arse diet'. One portion of steak and chips, followed by chocolate bread and butter pudding with ice cream.

'Doctor's orders' I say to the barmaid, who just smiles.

'Eat, eat and eat' had been the hospital's orders, 'build up the body fat before starting radiotherapy as you'll be losing your appetite then.'

Filling my face is exhausting, so time for a quick kip before Jess gets back, as we're out for dinner at Pizza Express (Mads is away on business tonight). Yet more 'wholesome' food: dough balls in butter, extra cheesy pizza, and chocolate fudge cake and ice cream, and the first glass of coke I've had in years.

Somehow cholesterol levels seem of minor relevance now.

We have a really nice father and daughter evening. It's great just chatting away with Jess about school, her mates, attitudes, what's happening. It's just a delight to see how she is growing up.

It's been a good first week back, and I even managed one twenty minute bike ride. It felt so good to get out and do something. What takes the most effort is trying to remain positive, particularly as there was a slight dip when I read in

Lance Armstrong's book something to the effect that if chemo doesn't work you've got about three months...

Best it works then!

Off to the dentist to check on his advice about pre-radiotherapy extractions and no surprise at all with his answer – one more to come out. Three in one hit all in different parts of the mouth. That should ensure I don't say much for a few hours, and could put a temporary halt on the calorie intake.

Meet up for another social with Robin and Chris for the 'cancer comparison' chat. It's a nice relaxing evening, but not much further insight into the treatment as Robin's chemo had been different, and he had an easy time with radio, interestingly though not losing his appetite, or having much trouble eating.

Life seems to be more normal now, even if, like a small child, I do need a sleep in the day, and I'm doing pretty much no exercise. I'm heeding hospital advice and eating like the proverbial pig, but not putting on any weight.

'New diet – get throat cancer, lose weight!' I daresay the marketing fraternity could come up with a more saleable strap-line.

Business as usual

Trying to keep the business ticking over, I'm pushing ahead with some business meetings this week and my new website, the latter being nearly ready to go live. I've also had a meeting with Gaynor and Heather of the Landirani Trust and started planning the entry to the Joan Wakelin Bursary Award, to try and win a commission to photograph the charity's work in Malawi for guaranteed coverage in The Guardian and The Royal Photographic Society.

81

We are chatting away when I notice a hard lump on my arm just below where the cannula had been for the chemo – it's a little swollen, red and sore to the touch so wound up the discussion, left, called the hospital to see what I should do, and was 'invited' back in.

'What is this lump in my arm?' I can't help but wonder. It seems to be getting larger, harder to the touch, redder, and is getting very sensitive.

Heading off for hospital I was trying hard to avoid the inevitable 'what if' thoughts, and was seen by Dr Disapproving, the doctor who had put me on 'withdrawal symptoms watch'. Yet more blood tests were carried out, and I was put on antibiotics for the lump, and told the 'there is good news and bad news'. The good was to say the white blood cell count was excellent (chemo often reduces this so lowering the usual defences of the body).

The bad was to say my kidney functionality had fallen, and would need attention to pick it up sufficiently to go through phase two of chemo next week. The remedy was no more tea, no more coffee, no alcohol, and at least three litres of water each day. Slight change of liquid intake then!

Back home I'm getting some positive comments from friends and neighbours. 'We think you're handling this really well, and our thoughts are with you' – nice to hear.

I smile to myself. *'Handling it well?'* Who knows? As far as I am concerned I'm just trying to ensure I've enough on my mind to avoid spending all day worrying about what will happen and the unknown.

Get them out!

It's time for another trip back to hospital to see the 'jolly' dentist and remove the three teeth. In spite of enough sedative to knock out an elephant, the first was so painful I made a few involuntary, though valiant, attempts to escape, but with no success. The second didn't want to come out at all so she applied plenty of 'extra muscle'. The noises coming from my mouth were not encouraging. The third and last was a relative breeze.

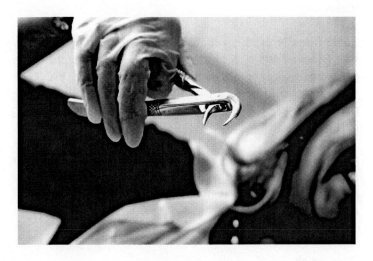

'Only three to pull.'

'You may have a little bruising from the second one', Liz calmly advised me – the master of the understatement. Or, as Anna rather quaintly put it when collecting me 'I wouldn't sit next to you on the train! It looks a little like you've been three rounds with Mike Tyson'.

I suspect the current 'eat, eat, and eat......' philosophy may be tricky for the next couple of days!

All things considered I was in good spirits, had taken Helen's advice and started the photo diary with the teeth-extraction torture tools. Back home Jess was heavily into rehearsals for

'Grease' where she had a big role playing Rizzo, including two solos, and I'm set up to do the photography.

I ended up taking over 700 shots at the dress rehearsal, thought the show was great, and thoroughly enjoyed doing the photography. I just got them delivered on time to the school before heading off to another networking session in Richmond.

Some friendly faces, including Helen, who commented how well I looked and how chirpy I seemed. Met Al, a customer, and started chatting about the forthcoming 'polo' event – I was supposed to be a part-sponsor with an exhibition stand, but wasn't going to be able to make it now, due to being hospitalised.

She then suggested I emailed her my photo, she would print and circulate it so there would be a number of 'Keith clones' running around! How really sweet of her: but is Richmond really ready for this?

Face-mask

I headed off on the now well-trodden route to hospital to check if the rather dull diet of three litres of water and no alcohol had had the correct effect on the kidneys, and to have the mould made for the facemask required for radiotherapy.

Once more into the depths of the Marsden after the inevitable blood tests, those now familiar white-walled rooms, and the no natural light.

'This won't hurt much' the nurse says with a sadistic smile, and her colleague grabs my arm and plunges this huge needle into, and seemingly straight through my arm. 'Get the strait-jacket'.

Perhaps one horror film too many in earlier years.

The nurses are fantastic and start covering my face, neck and shoulders in cream, followed by some blue stuff (a little like the material used for taking teeth moulds), and then some plaster of Paris. Also they were game on to take some photos so my latest 'adventure' had been well recorded.

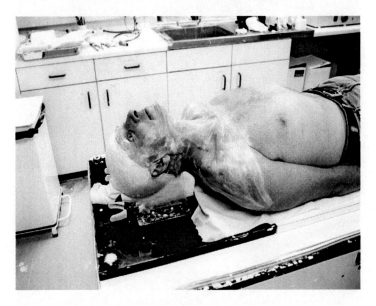

Mask-making stage 1.

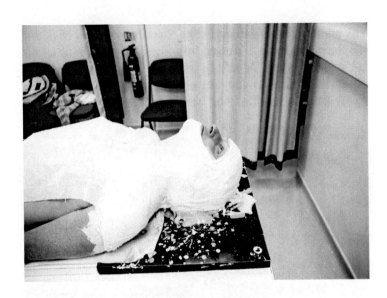

On with the plaster of Paris.

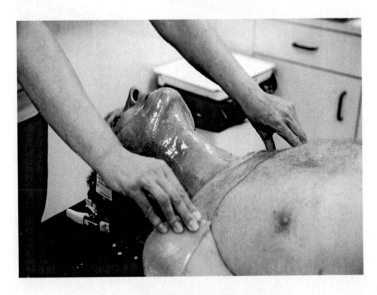

Looking good

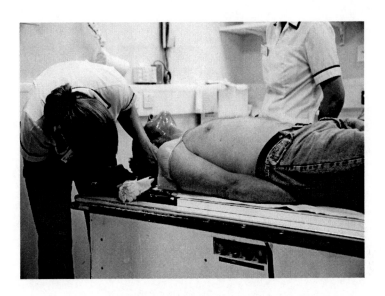

Check those measurements.

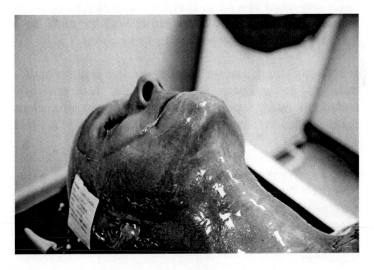

Skin tight fit.

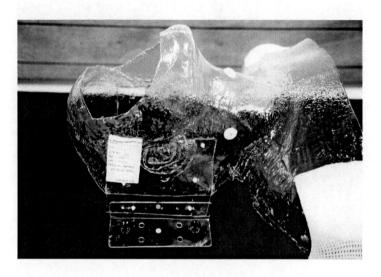

The finished article.

Back home Jess was only too happy to take my photo (she has a very good eye for a shot) and email that to Al along with the one taken three hours earlier with the mask on – leave her to decide which makes the better clone!

It's 'Grease' night, and we're off to see Jess strut her stuff – excellent performance (in my humble, and obviously completely neutral opinion she is brilliant), and all the kids really seemed as though they enjoyed themselves, plus I sold a good number of prints. All in all great fun.

Plus, I met a few other parents I haven't seen for a while. News of my condition had reached a few more than anticipated, but all were very complimentary on my appearance, and said there would be pints waiting for the 'father's beers' come the start of the girls' hockey season in September.

Back in soon – I can always look forward to more hospital food.

5. Face-off

Only two months have passed since being diagnosed – it feels longer as so much seems to have happened.

It's Monday 30th July and I'm in for pre-chemo blood tests (there is a top-up session in the first week of the radiotherapy), and the last radiotherapy planning session.

I had forgotten that this began with an EDTA test. I'm injected with some chromium and told to come back in three hours. Then they do another test to work out how the kidney functionality is, and what sort of extra boost may be required prior to the one hour chemo top-up that coincides with the start of radio on Thursday.

New language

Down to the depths again, this time it's off to radiotherapy for the training run, to be met by the same smiling nurse who remembered me from taking photos at the previous mask-fitting 'ceremony'. I was duly strapped down, the mask fitted and off through the machine – only a dummy-run as it's for x-rays to check all positions are correct.

The large cylindrical head starts rotating around my head, green lines appear on my face and neck – this is rather like playing an amusement-arcade laser game, except I'm the target and can't move!

The nurses have now switched and are speaking some alien dialect… it's 92–8, 94-6 or 96-4 – what's all that about then? Apparently the distance from the laser to the tumours needs to be 100 cms, and 94-6 represents 94 to the edge of the face and 6 from there to the tumour. The different numbers simply represent the measurements from the different angles from which I am going to be lasered.

As hospital visits go this was quite entertaining and relaxed, so I left with a smile, but will be back in for the serious stuff in no time.

Re-admitted

It's back to check-in at my now second home, The Royal Marsden, and the now familiar routine of a blood test, but the queue is too long so I'm sent off to radiotherapy straight away, for a last couple of scans with the mask fitted.

The nurse takes me off into a side room for 'a chat'. She re-states the list of the side-effects I'm likely to feel (they seem very keen to emphasise this rather grim aspect of the treatment), confirms the treatment timescales, emphasises that I can't smoke or drink spirits, and finishes with a bright and breezy 'any questions?'

It's time to be strapped down. But first an explanation into the machine noise (nothing like an MRI scan says the old hand), revolving x-ray unit, and therapy gun (mutually incompatible I would have thought?). 'The first circuit will be another test for x-rays only, then we will run a final check on the precise positions for the lasering' I was helpfully informed.

Lights off, machine on, and it starts revolving to reveal a ceiling picture of blue skies, sun and palm trees. 'Is this where they send me to recuperate?' I ask a little optimistically. 'Afraid not' was the all too predictable response.

The first two or three sessions will be with the full mask while they perfect their aim, then various sections of the mask are cut away in all the places I'm going to be lasered – apparently eleven different ones, so not just the two tumours.

It was explained that with Squamous cell cancer (the technical name for the type of cancer I have) they know exactly how, and where it would spread to, so knock out all those places as well as the tumours – seems like a good plan to me.

Now the routine is set for the next six weeks – sign in at reception, join the queue in the waiting room, and you'll be 'seen to' at the appointed time each day.

However, on the third day I'm kept in overnight for the first of two chemo top-ups – just the one hour of cisplatin this time. It's the same old routine though: kidney tests, more re-hydration prior to the chemo, middle of the night drip changes, but this time I'm back home after the next day's radiotherapy.

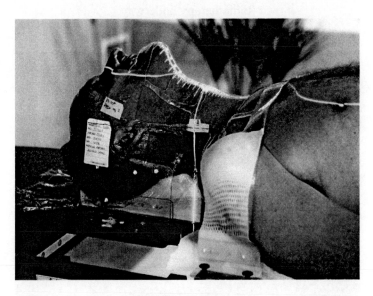

Precise targeting.

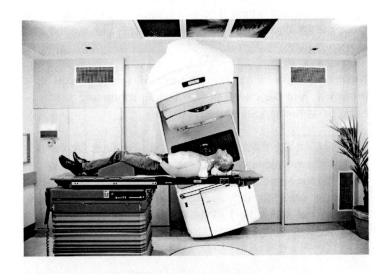

Radiotherapy underway.

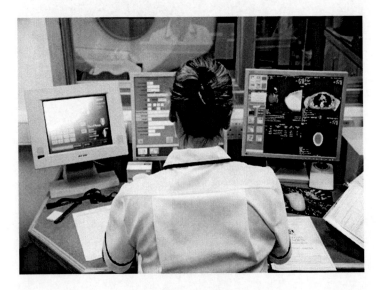

Mission control.

By that evening I am feeling truly dire – this is far worse than how I felt after the five days of chemo. I'm just lying on the settee feeling queasy, not wanting to eat, and thinking any minute I'm going to throw up.

I just about make it in to the hospital the next day, in dire need of some extra medication. Yet more anti-sickness pills are prescribed, but thankfully they do work very quickly, and very well. Back into line for my next microwaving session.

Looking around at my fellow sufferers in the queue I can't help but feel some of these guys look really sick. *'Will I look that bad in a couple of weeks?'*

After the first few days it's 'hi' as I walk in as the patient list is pretty similar so some faces are getting familiar, but this is not a social scene. Glum faces all round as the treatment is clearly taking its toll.

Each session only lasts about ten minutes and is a bit like going on a sun bed – at the end I just have this warm feeling all over my neck and shoulders.

'New' eating habits

After the first full week of radiotherapy it's off to Sussex to stay with my parents, and visit the 'chilli festival' at West Dean outside Chichester, now an annual event and chance to stock up on all those spicy sauces.

We arrived in time for lunch on the Saturday and were greeted by a spread of French bread, assorted cheeses and ham and salad. I dive in as I'm starving, but something's changed.

I am having trouble chewing, and swallowing is taking an age. It's not gone unnoticed that I am eating so slowly all of a sudden.

Come dinner, and the special fillet steak that Mum's made as a treat and I'm struggling, big time. Very small mouthfuls and as I'm endlessly chewing, the meat just seems to coagulate in my mouth, and makes me want to retch. I only just managed to finish the meal, and need to keep drinking just to get the food down.

The dry-mouth effect has begun - radiotherapy dries up the saliva so it's more difficult to break down any food, so chewing and swallowing are becoming difficult.

It looks like I've started out on that list of side effects.

Low spirits

It's Sunday and it's off to the chilli festival, normally a good excuse to try all these hot and spicy chilli sauces/beers/cheeses - anything! I can't handle the spices, nor eat much as it's all dry so I can't chew – a low mist of depression envelopes me – this is only after the first week, 25 more sessions to go.

'Oh how much worse is it going to get?'

Week two goes by uneventfully, except that by the end of it I have lost most of my taste, can't really chew at all and eating has become a real problem. So my staple diet has pretty much become soup, cereal, yoghurt, smoothies, custard and mineral water.

Everything has started to taste the same, a bit like cardboard and become distinctly unappealing. As a result I am now losing energy, feeling tired and starting to lose weight.

Week three, and the trip up to the hospital has become a real task, walking up the steps at Wimbledon and South Kensington tube stations is now a real effort and very tiring,

94

and my general mental state of mind is going downhill rapidly as I know I'm not even halfway through the radiotherapy.

Nothing's easy now, everything tiring.......

Ray of light

Always keeping half an eye open for an opportunity I had of course handed out business cards to any of the hospital staff that had the dubious pleasure of dealing with me.

One of the radiographers came up and gleefully said he'd looked at my website www.keithhern.com, seen the link to londonphotos.com and couldn't believe it but his sister was best mates at school with one of the daughters of the other photographer featured on the site. Small world!

A welcome distraction from my deteriorating state, this was a good excuse for a chat about photography, and the associated general improvement in my spirits (I eventually met up with his sister in the following March for an amusing chat about the world of freelance photography).

Back to the daily drudge of joining the queue of glum faces.

I'm about half way through the radiotherapy, and I joined the depressing queue as usual, my face no doubt as glum as all the others, but today would be different.

All of a sudden amongst this line of long faces a cheerful face appeared, a young lady with a huge smile, friendly demeanour and a mate to accompany her. We got chatting and she had managed to find a friend to chaperone her when coming up and down to hospital for treatment.

'God it's so good to see a smiling face' was my first thought, and she had an immediate impact on my state of mind. We

started chatting and got on really well. Mel is from South London, working down the road from me in Kingston. Her arrival completely changed my outlook to the daily visits – now I looked forward to seeing her each day, and whatever mate had been recruited as her latest chaperone.

Curiosity got the better of me after a couple of days and I asked what 'brand' she had. 'I've already had it removed from the middle of my head' she said nonchalantly. I winced at the thought, before saying 'go on'...

She swept back her long blonde hair.

'See that?' she said revealing a scar that went from below one ear, up and all round her head down to below her other ear.

Cringing a little I asked 'so what happened?'

'They found the tumour in the middle of my head so had to open my head up, peel my face off, break my jaw, surgically remove the tumour, re-set my jaw, pull my face back up and stitch it in place!'

Momentarily I was stunned into silence while I took all that in.

'Oh my God, but you look absolutely amazing'. A very pretty lady anyway, even more so considering what she'd been through. I felt like I was having a stroll in the park by comparison. We became friends and would cheer each other up as the next few weeks went by – Mel had just started when we met, so I was some three weeks ahead and well-placed to outline in detail all (or so I thought) of the 'delightful' side effects, she had to come.

Taste – what's that?

By now everything tastes of cardboard, I haven't eaten anything requiring chewing for ten days or so, have had no wine or beer (normally an integral part of my 'balanced' diet), am shedding weight at an amazing rate, and have virtually no energy at all. It's tough now, everything is a major effort.

I wonder what the world looks like for the consultant. Another normal day at the office for him. He's a bit behind schedule, probably grateful that it's just Keith Hern and two more patients before it's back home. Bet his wife is a great cook, and he's thinking about that cold beer before dinner. Maybe he's even hungry already and speculating on what will be served at home.

Andrew arrives for my check-up, asks a few questions, spends longer than usual looking at my mouth, sticks the camera up my nose and down the back of my throat, pronounces all is going well, and asks how the side effects are. I explain in detail and he nods knowingly, simply stating that is exactly what was expected and don't worry they'll be monitoring progress.

So all the gloomy predictions at the start were coming true.

As luck would have it Anna was in a position to drive me to and from the hospital. The lifts were very much appreciated, though I don't suppose I was much in the way of company.

I'm trying very hard to stay in a good frame of mind, but it's becoming a real test now, and looming large is my last chemo session in week five of radiotherapy. Can't say that's something I'm looking forward to, after how I felt after the first top-up session.

What's not helping is the knowledge that, even when treatment finishes, the side effects get worse as the effects of the treatment are cumulative so I'm likely to be suffering for most/all of September, and it's only the second half of August!

Mentally I'm struggling.......

6. Round Two

Check-in

Going back to the second round of chemotherapy, just like getting a flight I need to check in early.

'The hospital is so full' said the chap on reception 'that you will be in the main ward rather than that side-room before'. Not a huge difference, but it made me even more appreciative of the medical insurance Mads has through her work.

Anyway, first stop is the basement to fit the radiotherapy mask – it's made out of transparent plastic for the laser treatment that's to come. All fitted fine, and more of the nurses game on for taking photos – a hospital full of budding photographers. Now it's off for the next CAT scan complete with facemask.

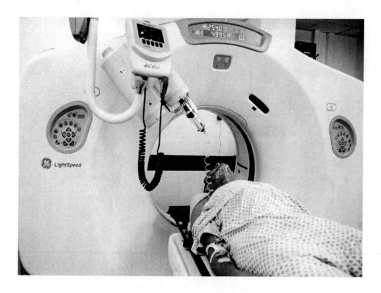

Alignment okay?

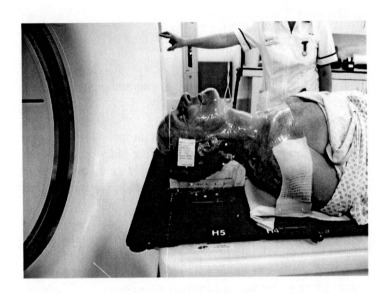

Here goes.

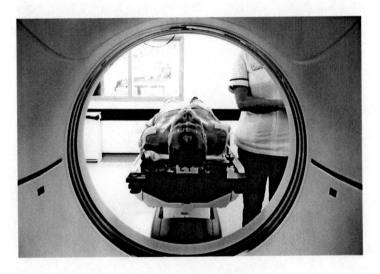

'View' from the other side.

Same old routine, another cannula, an iodine injection, then into the scanner – fortunately another nurse happy to take the shots. She seemed to enjoy it so much maybe she's going to swap career. I am very grateful to all the medical staff who helped out with the photography – thank you! Scan duly done, so off up to have the permanent cannula fitted for the chemo – it's a bit like being a pin-cushion again today.

It's back to the ward, with my three other 'inmates', all of whom seemed a little worse off than me. The guy on the right had a visit from his wife – 'there are no spuds at home', 'come to that we're out of food', 'now I'm going to have to go shopping' – on and on she went, just the kind of moral support the man needed when he's got cancer. Wouldn't be surprised if he volunteered to be retained for longer to avoid going back to that nagging!

Diagonally opposite me is an Asian gent who didn't look in a good way at all. He was feeding himself through a stomach tube, and having to lean over every so often and cough up god knows what into a bucket! Opposite was empty to start with, but soon filled by a gent with a nasal tube who had trouble speaking and was depositing phlegm into a plastic cup whenever required.

Sound effects in this ward are not the most attractive!

Time for a walk round and check out who else is around. I saw the lady who was in the next room to me last time – she hadn't been home! I stopped for a chat. She was looking much better than before and was strongly suggesting I buy some 'Aqueous Cream' and start using it now on my neck, in preparation for the radiotherapy. I made a mental note to check out the medical advice on this.

101

Liquid intake

Mads has arrived, so we go for a walk, and get a coffee. It tastes good after a few days without.

Some less good news from her work. Her boss, who seemed so thoughtful to start with, is now kicking up a fuss about her spending time in hospital with me, as it's affecting her work. He wants her to take some leave.

Not very thoughtful would be an understatement. She's got enough in the way of concerns at the moment, and being able to at least continue working gives her something to think of other than my situation. Odd how people change their tune, but I guess we are getting used to that now.

There's no stopping that corporate juggernaut, and its continuous drive for growth and profits. No time for trivia like your husband is in hospital being treated for a life-threatening condition. That might even put her boss's no doubt substantial bonus at risk, and that clearly can't be allowed to happen.

Dr Disapproving arrives, does a quick MOT (pulse, heart, breathing, stomach pains) and gives me an 'all working well' rating, except the kidney functionality is still down, so will put me on saline drip for four hours to re-hydrate.

A familiar-sounding voice starts, before the culprit's even arrived at my bedside 'now what's all this I hear, you're not drinking enough?' says Sue. 'Oh oh in trouble again' I reply smiling. She's such a nice lady. Apparently one of the effects of cisplatin and 5FU is dehydration so I need to force more liquid down all the time.

'You must try harder', she says, bringing back ghastly memories of such comments scattered across old school reports. Sue hints I'll be moved back to the same room as before in the morning – can't say I'm sad about that! She confirms that and after breakfast I'm back in solitary. Great!

Good news comes in that the test results are fine so chemo round two starts this evening.

There is the usual cosmopolitan mixture of nurses, the most intriguing being the lady from Barbados, also interested in travel, having just been to Rome, but interestingly with a husband who is retired and spends half his life in Barbados. He seems to have life well sorted out.

'So half of the time you are a ten-hour flight away from your husband?' I commented, just checking I had understood. 'Not a problem' she replies 'makes for a successful marriage'. I'm less convinced.

Time to be 'switched on' again, linked up for the saline drip at 7 p.m. so it's 11 p.m. for the anti-vomit, 11.30 for the cisplatin, 12.30 for the flush through, then finally at 1 a.m the 5FU. And maybe some sleep!

Saturday morning brings a power cut, so I'm weighed by wheelchair this morning – never did really understand the link!

'So what happens if the power is off long enough for the battery on the drip to run out?' I enquire.

'The batteries are normally okay. Except when they're not.' came the carefully considered reply.

'That's okay then – no need to worry' I said to the nurse who just realised what she had said, so both had a laugh. How good that feels, and I still notice whenever it happens – it's the little things.

To add to the faces and nationalities previously met, in strolled another new nurse (or at least new to me). This time from Trinidad and Tobago so we swapped tales about sipping a rum punch at Pigeon Point whilst rocking gently in a hammock. How good does that sound!

Cream cakes and 'The Secret'

A very old friend suddenly appeared, and had clearly been well-briefed as he was bearing gifts of cream cakes – they should help the expanding waistline. Chocolate éclairs – years since I've had one of those, and don't they taste good!

Wake up the next morning and for the first time since all this started I feel sick, and I don't think it's from one too many an éclair! I mention this to the nurse, and it's another step up in medication levels. The mounting number of pills I'm on is getting to be an impressive list.

Now it's time to focus the mind and watch this much-vaunted 'The Secret'. In the NLP world of all things mental, anyone I've come across has mentioned this book in the hushed tones of extreme reverence......so....

The thousands of years old 'Secret' turns out to be within me, you, everyone – merely a case of working out how use it. The CD features many a rich individual, all of whom seem to have successfully harnessed the power of positive thought to turn their lives around into achieving all they want.

One person after another proudly stating how they've harnessed 'the Secret' to achieve their five houses, four boats, six first class holidays a year, or whatever has been their life's ambition.

It won't be to everyone's taste, but I am certainly left reflecting that there must be something in this 'positive mental thought' process, so merely re-enforcing the thoughts from the work done with Helen.

Italy – on or off?

The next treatment break is getting close, just a few days away now, but it's getting tight, the diary is cluttered, is this at risk?

Right now it's Monday 16th July, I'm due out of here on Wednesday, back for an MRI scan on Thursday, and off to Italy on Friday for a week – no room for slippage if I'm to make that plane.

The diary remains 'full' as I'm back from Italy on the 28th July, in on the 30th for another follow-up CT scan and radiotherapy prep session, kick off the radiotherapy on August 2nd, finish September 13th, plus the two top-up chemo sessions, so there are a few questions for the doc tomorrow.

Top of the priority list – Italy, will it still be okay?

It has to be okay. This has been my first major mid-treatment marker point.

In come the medics – I have fingers crossed a little nervously. 'You've put on a few kilos and there has been a slight rise in your blood pressure' is the statement. Very little else is said. I reckon this is just a reaction to 'what if they say I can't go'.

Time for the late evening tests and they're okay – it's looking good.

I have a new next door neighbour this morning, and he's well down track from me, and soon to be 'released'. He was in for an op to remove his tumour after three chemo sessions and thirty five radiotherapy, and he didn't look bad at all, in comparison to his predecessor.

We were chatting away, when he explained his diagnosis, which was extraordinary. Having been sent back home after fracturing a shoulder working in Italy he'd gone to see his doctor to check on progress on the shoulder. Whilst there he asked him to check out a small lump he'd recently found on his neck.

The doctor started feeling the shoulder and after a couple of minutes looked him straight in the eyes.

The only words the doctor said were 'oh shit!' Nothing else – with that succinct medical summation the diagnosis was known and his worst nightmare had just started. We swapped stories about how diagnosis results in instant mental meltdown, and just how terrifying those first few hours and days are.

I did ask a few questions about radiotherapy. He said he had no problem through the treatment, but afterwards some discomfort and the small matter of radiation burns on the inside of his mouth.

I couldn't help but notice, in complete contrast to the 'previous' tenant his neck wasn't in the slightest bit red or burnt, so asked what cream he'd used as this looked so much better.

He'd used the highly recommended Radiance Cream from the Bristol (Penny Brohn) Cancer Centre rather than the Aqueous cream used by the previous incumbent.

First job when I get back – buy a job lot of Radiance Cream.

The medics and Italy

A seemingly endless mini-stream of visitors was coming and going now.

'Would I get involved in another clinical trial and have weekly CT scans throughout radiotherapy?' 'Sure' I said,

106

guessing that if anything untoward should happen that would enhance the chance of detection.

'Stay calm, it'll be okay, you'll be in Italy soon' I'm telling myself. It's my release day, so I can go walkabout in the morning, and get back for the MRI later... Anna's around so should even have another photo assistant!

In comes Doctor Disapproving (is the withdrawal watch lady going to scupper the trip?).

'What about Italy? I wanted to scream at her.

As if reading my mind she started, 'As for Italy', she has my undivided attention. 'It's looking very good now, we'll give you the requisite cancer card, associated letter, and antibiotic prescription just in case the thrombiotic bumps (that lump on my arm needing antibiotics) re-appear.' Fantastic! I'm on that plane.

She continued 'The biggest risk is an infection on the plane – we will check your white blood cell count on Wednesday, but I figure you are really looking forward to this so unless there is a last-minute problem you can go!' She smiled obviously appreciating how important the trip is to me. Dr. Disapproving - she's not so bad after all.

'Can't wait – mentally I'm on that plane now, I just love it out there, the food, the wine, the scenery, the relaxed way of life....'

A couple of friends appeared with a bag full of extremely smelly cheese. Might just be dinner when I'm home tomorrow with the first glass of wine for two weeks! Got to do some last minute practice for the Italian diet!

I'm woken up at one to have the chemo switched off, and was so pleased to have got through phase two I didn't get back to sleep until five, so will be absolutely shattered later, but who cares?

It's crunch time. The medical entourage are due to go through final questioning about Italy, medication, hospital and flight notes.

Fred, the teetotal Irish Charge Nurse just popped by to say hi and that he's really looking forward to going uptown on his day off tomorrow. Chinatown for lunch followed by the Harry Potter movie. Certainly want to go and see that myself soon, it's one of those Dad and daughter treats (for me more than Jess probably!).

The entourage are coming - the doctor just pops his head round the door, and cheerily says Italy is all cleared.

Perfect!

The priest

He's around again. I'd seen the priest wandering the wards on a couple of occasions now.

It may well be that patients have deep-seated religious beliefs, or possibly priests as friends, but to me it meant there could be some 'last rites' being administered. It's a stark reminder that not everyone gets to walk out of here. The goose bumps make a brief re-appearance.

Travel orders

Back home and now I need to sleep before the early start to Italy on Friday. Like a kid about to go on holiday, I can't wait. My first day back was spent sprawled in front of the TV watching the first day of The Open golf – dozing and watching, and just planning how to get enough sleep on the way to Elba tomorrow.

Sorted, I think: sleep on the motorway to Stansted (we have to leave at 5 a.m.), then on the plane, in the car from Pisa, on the ferry to Elba and then hopefully should be okay for the trip. This worked a treat and we arrived at the hotel some thirteen hours after leaving home, but feeling good and really looking forward to a break.

'*Do not to drink very much, but eat as much as you can and whatever you like*' were my dietary instructions. Better listen this time. However I remained in blissful ignorance of the forthcoming effects of radiotherapy.

Elba turned out to be a fantastic place to visit, with plentiful good little restaurants, excellent scenery and weather, not quite enough to keep two teenage girls fully interested, but they managed to get along (just!).

The dietary advice was heeded for at least the first couple of days, but then the temptation of all that nice wine to accompany the excellent food was too much, so over-indulged on both fronts for the remainder of the trip.

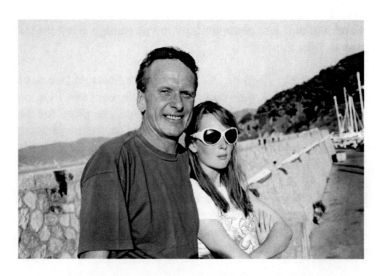

With Jess in Elba for the mid-treatment break.

'This is my mid-treatment break after all, so must make the most of it. Too much good red wine here not to indulge. And anyway who knows what the radiotherapy will bring when I get home?' – had no problem justifying my excesses.

The calm before the storm?

Back to the mainland and our regular place, Colleoli, twenty minutes from Pisa for four good relaxing days in the summer sunshine.

Another excellent trip to Italy is coming to an end – I'm getting addicted to this country, it really does get better with every visit. All that pasta, prosciutto e formaggio, wild boar, bruschetta, all washed down with a few glasses of local 'grape juice' – obviously within the medically-advised limits.

'Will I be okay to enjoy the next trip in November?' was on my mind as we set off for Pisa airport.

Radiotherapy, those dire warnings. That long list of side effects. Can't say I'm looking forward to getting back.

7. Medical Testing and Dire Warnings.

Mentally, for some reason, I've just rolled back to the early days at the beginning of treatment, and the first operation.

Under the knife

Mads and I arrive at St. Anthony's well in time, and I'm trying very hard to stay relaxed, but failing miserably. Having never been 'admitted' before I was blissfully ignorant of the need to appear hours before anything is going to happen, something that still remains a mystery.

An hour and half relaxing before John Timothy (the consultant surgeon) turns up to explain exactly what he's going to do, but he starts by dropping a casual, almost throw-away comment. 'By the way, the scan results are through, and the cancer is localised.'

'So?' I wanted to hear more. This is the first piece of really good news, and confirms I have only two tumours, one in my neck and the other in my throat. Nothing else!

'So', he continued, 'that means we know the extent of your cancer and it hasn't spread anywhere else. The primary tumour, as I suspected, is not the lump on your neck, but is hidden away under the surface of the skin on the back of your tongue, and was exceedingly difficult to spot – impossible to find without the PET scan.'

He has a very relaxed and confident style of explaining what he will be doing, which does help my nerves. I'm listening intently as he carefully explains how he's going to sedate me and then operate to remove the bulk of the primary tumour, and also undertake various other biopsies around my mouth, the results of which will be known within about a week.

'I'll see you in theatre in a little while, in the meantime we'll send the anaesthetist round to tell you what he's going to do, and then you'll be collected by a porter and taken to the operating room'.

'Breathe this oxygen in and then we'll operate, it'll only take about 40 minutes.' A couple of breaths later and the room is spinning (I may have come across that feeling before in my life, but never due to gas inhalation).

The next thing I know, I'm in recovery. Back to my room, and see Mads, all is fine, surgeon has already spoken to her and said I'm a pretty fit man. Always nice to hear, even if now I feel anything but.

News of my situation was spreading like wildfire as numerous phone calls came in that evening from friends and relatives.

As the saying goes 'you only find out who your real friends are when you need them.' Guess I'll be finding that out over the next few months. 'Be ready for some surprises on that count, in both ways' was what I had heard. Time will tell.

Exchanged a few hi-tech messages with Jess at home, and even found out how to send a live voice message. That is progress for such a technophobe. I am very aware of her situation, but have no idea at all how it must feel as a fourteen year old to know your Dad has been diagnosed with something that could kill him. How will her school friends react? She'd been gossiping with her mates for over an hour – situation normal, but they all seem very supportive as well.

Madeleine came to collect me to go home, weighed down by the vast number of painkillers in case there was a reaction to the op and the throat started to play up.

The first of the numerous hospital visits had been completed successfully.

Next stop

My personal hospital tour shifts to the Royal Marsden in Fulham where I am sent to get the low-down on treatment from the consultant who would be running all my chemotherapy and radiotherapy treatment.

Arrival involved the completion of seemingly endless regulatory forms, followed by an introduction to a nurse who just wanted to take a 'nose swab'.

'Just checking to see if you are going to bring along MRSA with you or not' she advises cheerfully before sticking said swab up my nose.

'Fine', I replied, a little less cheerful at the prospect than she was!

Lead consultant

Andrew Jones was to be my consultant – seemed to be really professional and very pleasant. My first impressions of the two consultants I have could not be better.

In what is fast becoming the standard first step on each hospital visit he stuck that funny camera up my nose and down the back of my throat again still feels strange, however he assures me I'll get used to it as he'll do it every time he sees me. Great!

Leaning back in his chair he slowly removes his glasses, looks at me with a serious-looking expression, before embarking on a long list of how traumatic this will be for the body, just how grim I'm going to feel, why and when. All delivered in that matter-of-fact, no frills style of the medical world – with all the subtlety of a sledgehammer.

'Any questions?' he asks.

Somewhat dumbstruck by this gruesome sounding list, and feeling my spirits tumbling, about all I can manage is a less than confident:

'When can we get started?'

Then through this haze of traumas, side effects, and generally how absolutely shit I will be feeling remember one more important, make that 'vital', point that must be covered.

'And what chance will we have of keeping the week's holiday in Italy booked for the end of July?'

'We will start soon, and leave it with me, but the holiday may well be possible. What will you do now?' asks Andrew, 'go and have a drink' I respond. 'Sounds like a good plan to me' says he. *'What a decent guy'.*

I've got a session booked with Helen in the morning – fixed in case I need support if the hospital news was bad. It hadn't been, so headed off in good spirits and wondering what direction I'll be taken in the next 'head session'.

'Tell me about your week, are you still being visited by the gremlins?' Sort of. Covered the tears in the car incident, how the surgeon said he'd taken more biopsies. Had a negative turn when the bulk of the tumour had been removed and suddenly read this as implying more problems and uncertainty. The treatment has only just begun and my mind is all over the place. One minute positive about getting through it, the next more like 'is this it?'

Strangely though at this moment I'm feeling positive, but aware this is a mindset I will need to build on.

'How do you feel?'

'Fine, positive at this moment, just have this thought that something is happening I'm not sure I can explain, which is kind of weird'...

'Go on' she encourages. 'It's just I really didn't expect I'd feel like this two/three weeks after being diagnosed with cancer' I try to explain. 'And this 'mind stuff' I'm finding really helpful when it comes to coping'. Coping may be an exaggeration, but at least it's helping me to focus on the upside, as the alternative really is grim!

'You have made major steps already. Last time I saw you, you were all 'I want to do this, I have to do this, how can you help me make the necessary changes? And it was all from the head. Today it's from the heart, not the head – in other words what you are 'really' feeling, as opposed to what you want to feel.

'So what next?' she asks.

'Not sure, I feel like I've just set off to somewhere new, don't know where, nor how to get there, nor what will be there, but I'm on for the ride. Almost like an awakening or even enlightenment.' She just repeated those two words slowly and left them hanging.

'My task as a coach is to assist you with your own development, not specifically guide you at all, and you seem to be progressing fine so let's just catch up on a couple of other bits and pieces. How was the CD?' I covered my cynicism towards hypnotherapy, but said I'd found this quite easy to use, and very helpful. I related what the CD was about and said I'd used 'Jessica' as my keyword.

'When you look at her when do you see her?'

'In about four months i.e. when my treatment is finished'.

'Interesting', says she, 'why not when she's 50 or 60?'

Little remarks, that's all.

A different way of viewing things, delivered as ever in such a simple way for maximum impact. The underlying message is always the same - focus on a successful outcome, not the obstacles that you will come across en route.

As ever I left the session feeling much more upbeat.

'36'

Just realised I've only needed one of that mountain of painkillers I left hospital with, which must be good news.

Off to try 36 holes of golf with my brother-in-law as my partner. As instructed only three days after 'a general' (anaesthetic) the advice was take an electric trolley or buggy to ensure I'm not trying to do too much.

Opting for the former in the morning, it's first time I've ever used one like that, and quite likely to be the last. Far from being easy and relaxing it reminded me of the first time I drove a car - one minute hurtling off down the fairway as it's gone into overdrive, the next moment I'm holding tight only to find it heading for the deepest jungle in the wilds of Wimbledon.

I'm not on great form either, and had a falling out with my putter, which was sorted with a couple of re-shaping exercises across the knee as yet another straight ten inch putt never threatened to touch the hole. Mads would not be impressed– *'it's only a stupid game'* I can hear her saying.

Anyway, I finally finished the round and gleefully returned the aforementioned contraption with a mind of its own, headed for the 19th and some well-earned refreshment. The lunch at this event is always fantastic. A massive seafood platter, vast selection of cold meats and salads, sweets, cheeses, and normally accompanied by rather too much wine. This year it's a very restrained lunch on the liquid side, so picked up the afternoon set of wheels sober, although did manage to eat a mountain of food.

'For how much longer?'

Andrew Jones' long list of forthcoming 'delights' I think was the cause for my 'you won't be able to eat like this soon' approach to the lunch.

Actually, I felt a complete fraud using the buggy as I was fine, but I'm under instructions to 'take it easy'. I did get a few strange looks as a lot of the guys didn't know my condition, and just the one comedian, who upon seeing my new transport politely enquired: 'so when did you turn 70 then?'

It's odd, I reflect, just how important 'humour' has become, and how much more I notice the light-hearted moments.

It's the little things in life......

Normality?

Timesonline have been in touch again. 'There's been a change of plan and your Kenya piece won't be in the next edition. But don't worry, it'll be in the one following'. Years of sales meant I never did like the sound of these 'plan changes', but they were true to their word!

This could be an interesting evening as I'm off for my first networking event since diagnosis – and all in all feeling pretty good, considering.

I had planned to stop off at Helen's on the way, duly arrived, rang the bell and waited.

'Can't help but wonder what this feels like from her side of the door. Is she anxious, worried about how I'm coping. Or curious to see how a sceptic like me is reacting to the CD. Maybe she's going out later and just hoping I'm on time.'

'How are you? Still handling everything okay? You look fine.'

'Fine thanks, but had a big dip yesterday when I got the call that I'm due in next week for the start of the chemo.'

'How close does that feel?'

I put my hand up about a foot from my face – 'that close'.

'Do that again.' I dutifully follow instructions, and she simply moves my hand to the right a few inches. *'Now what do you see?'* 'Loads more, there's nothing in the way'. I answered, a little bemused.

'Focus on the positive, look round, over, under, or through whatever the problem is, but not on it.' So easy to say: not always so easy to do.

I left Helen in a good frame of mind, and walked into the networking group, immediately finding a friend from another such session who was stunned when I told her my news.

It's strange now, weird even, I seem to be getting used to telling people 'I've just been diagnosed with cancer'. It somehow doesn't seem quite as scary as it was. I'm even getting to the stage where watching the reaction is quite intriguing, as everyone reacts differently. I can almost see them thinking *'what shall I say now? Bad luck? You'll be fine? Try not to worry?'*. Come to think of it I'm not sure I'd know what to say – odd!

There are no preparations for the mental side of being diagnosed with the big 'C'.

The next morning I was doing the normal email updates when a message arrived from a lady I had met for the first time the previous evening, ' It was great to meet you, and what an inspiration you are the way you are handling your condition. Oh, and I love your photography.' I must be doing something right, but it certainly doesn't feel inspirational – more a case of get on with it as best I can.

Now it's off to Hampton Court for an early game of real tennis. It's only a few minutes up the road but long enough for the mind to go walkabout. *'When will I be able to play again after this morning? What if I can't? What is going to happen to me?'*

I don't seem able to keep the cancer out of my thoughts for long – maybe it's the impending chemotherapy.

I'm up against an Irish property developer whom I'd met a few times before – always worth a laugh and joke, a competitive game and the occasional cry of frustration as another potential winner rockets into the foot of the net.

Toyed with the idea of dropping the 'c' word before we started but thought that might be construed as gamesmanship, so left that until afterwards. We were having the usual after match chat with the pro, when I just said 'not sure when the next time I'll see you will be, I'm in hospital next week to start treatment for throat cancer, which will keep me out for at least six months'.

His jaw just fell open and he was speechless for a second or two. 'But you look fine. Anyway, all the best for a speedy recovery and look forward to another game when you've recovered.'

'Look fine…… and how long will that last?'

Something about his remark struck a chord.

119

On the outside, everything looks fine, it's the areas that you can't see that have the problems – where the tumours are, and of course the mind and the now daily turmoil that it goes through. I guess these must be the same feelings experienced by anyone diagnosed with something life-threatening, not just cancer... AIDS, MS, Parkinson's – it's what can't be seen by the naked eye.

No-one knows looking at you!

His comments made me aware of another aspect of what I had experienced to date - the kindness of people I know, or have met, is somewhat of a revelation. I don't know what I would have expected, but the extent of the kind comments, plus the numerous offers of assistance, are well... humbling is probably the best way of summing it up.

The learning experience continues.

Work

An old friend is coming round. She rang to ask if I'd do some portrait shots of her. No problem. A couple of hours and a few hundred shots later and we had a really good range of images.

The whole area of portrait photography remains fascinating to me. No matter how confident and attractive someone is, when you point a camera at them all of a sudden there's a different person.

As I've been told before 'You're a photographer – that's what you do, make me look good.' If only it were that simple.

I remember reading an article by a famous portrait photographer who described in meticulous detail how he would arrange his studio beforehand, set the scene, spend some time putting the subject at ease then fire off two 36 exposure films (yep, real photography as the die-hards would say) to start with. He hadn't loaded the film into the camera, but his experience told him that it would take that long before his subject would stand any chance of relaxing, and until that happened he had no chance of getting a decent shot. That always makes me feel better!

She listened to my 'recent history' but raised an eyebrow to 'finding the cancerous lump on my neck was an absolute godsend' so I explained that without finding that lump I would not have been diagnosed until the primary grew to such a size that… let's not go down that route'.

Back home we're planning something very unusual tonight – going out and celebrating our fifteenth wedding anniversary. Mads and I have long since stopped the usual birthday, Christmas, anniversary and Valentine's presents, in favour of putting the equivalent cash towards something we really enjoy – travelling.

This time though, it's different. *'Isn't everything these days'.* We're off to try a new fish restaurant in Cobham, and Jess has even said she'll come with us (teenage speak for haven't had a better offer, but it's great that she's happy to come along). Maybe in the back of her mind is the same thought that's in the back of mine – how long until we can do this again? Or will we be able to?

No matter how hard I try the 'c' word is never far from my thoughts…and the recurring theme - what does the future hold?

Another business meeting, this time with a new PR contact. She used to be a top-class swimmer, who ended up in bed for ten years unable to move (I can't recall what the condition was called) and now gets around in a wheelchair, but is also capable of standing for short periods and walking short distances.

I feel like I've only got a minor ailment by comparison to what she's been through.

There are plenty of people carrying on their lives with various illnesses, complaints – everyone is normally too busy to notice, or be concerned about, other people's problems. Funny how I notice this so much more now I've joined the ranks of 'the affected'.

The now normal evening taxi service is required to and from a singing lesson as Jess starts to get her solos ready for the school production of Grease, on 11th and 12th July. I really hope I can attend but there is a risk I will be back in hospital for chemo round two. Same risk with that holiday to Italy at the end of July. It's impossible to plan much at present.

I'm meeting up for an early evening pint at the local with my oldest mate (we've been good friends for approaching 35 years), and I haven't seen him for a while, but know he's got his own issues what with separating from his wife of some 18 years or so. All seems very amicable at present, but with two daughters aged between 8 and 13 it may not be easy once it comes to him actually moving out, which is due in a couple of weeks. It's nice evening having a quiet pint down the local with an old friend '*how long*?'

There it is again.

Next morning I head off for a game of golf with a 'bye love, see you later' as I close the front door behind me. The recurring thought for everything at present replays in my head again '*how long until the next one?*' it's getting louder and louder, the closer I get to the chemo that starts next week.

Most people now know my situation, but not everyone. One of the guys in the four ball game, upon hearing my news, simply stated 'I'm sorry to hear that. A friend of mine's other half has got cancer, she's just picked up an infection in hospital and as a result will be dead within ten days'. Everything suddenly feels cold.

'Why thanks for those words of encouragement – ever thought of a new career in PR?' Just staggering how someone intelligent could be so totally thoughtless: I'm fast reaching the conclusion that reactions and comments like this shouldn't come as a surprise any more, yet somehow they still do. And the immediate result is another wave of negative thoughts, the 'what ifs?'

The next day, a bright and sunny Sunday morning started with a bike ride with Mads. We'd only started cycling a couple of years ago, after she had come back from work one day and said she fancied doing the London-Brighton cycle race. Questioning her sanity at the time I should have known better, but if she was going to do it, so was I. After various amounts of training we had duly completed the 52 miles in a none-too-racy six hours last year.

Talking of charity events, it is strange to think that only three or four weeks ago I was watching Jess compete in 'Run for Life', a cancer event for those suffering, or who had lost friends and/or relatives to the disease.

I remember only too well reading the emotional messages on the back of the pink t-shirts worn by the vast majority of the runners. The timing of this couldn't have been more poignant for me coming, as it did, after my first set of tests, but before I'd had the results.

Every 'in loving memory of' message made me shiver involuntarily – was that going to be what fate had in store for me? No more than a message on Jess' back?

Jess is up when we return from the ride and has bought me a 'Fathers' Day' present – a DVD to keep me entertained in hospital, so sweet!

Keith who?

I called round to Helen to drop back the two other Suzi Smith hypnotherapy CDs. I had listened to part of the curiously entitled 'Communicating with Your Symptoms' - strange, long, and I just couldn't get my head around what was going on, so I'll save that for when I'm being chemo'd next week.

I'm subdued. The proximity of the treatment is starting to have its effect, but Helen's great as usual and we just chat. I mention I'm writing a diary. It started off as a dumping ground for my mental turmoil that followed 'that' phone call, a way to remain sane, but then I just continued. Who knows, maybe I can get it published?

Listening with interest, a broad smile breaks out across her face, and she just says: 'with the greatest respect, who the hell is Keith Hern? It's not as though you're famous so who is going to buy the book? Why not do what you are good at, and do a photo diary of the treatment, as I'm not aware of anything like that existing'. Neat idea - I'll do it.

I will arrange for another 'head' session, as I've come to call the work with Helen, after round one of chemo, but if I need to I can call her which is cool. I head for home armed with some new scientific reading material. Dr. Bruce Lipton's 'The Biology of Belief' and 'Molecules of Emotion' by neuroscientist Candace Pert PhD. Madeleine really is starting to query my sanity now!

Back home, a quick burst of Suzi Smith, and a mid-afternoon knock on the door from a neighbour. Fancy a glass of wine? He knows us far too well. It's such a sociable street, it's great. Mads and I go round for a glass or two (I'm obviously trying to be restrained with impending hospital tests tomorrow), and it sounds like I may have some visitors whilst I'm 'hotelling' it in the Royal Marsden.

I wonder how many will drop by when I'm in hospital? Real friends?

Back again, and another knock on the door. One of the other neighbours has a birthday so it's the standard glass or two of champagne. This is starting to test my (not so great) willpower of restraint. I keep it to another glass and a half to stay within reasonable limits, and return home over an hour later having kept consumption down to about three glasses overall – a good effort!

In the thirty yards or so to the front door I can feel my state of mind is rapidly changing – what is this chemotherapy treatment going to be like? Just how dire will it make me feel?

Sleeping is a problem. All I seem to think of is Andrew's comments about how traumatic this will be for my body, and how dreadful I'll feel.

Sweet dreams!

8. Secondaries

The treatment finished weeks ago, the body will have calmed down enough for the all-important check-up. Has the treatment worked?

It is now just days away, and the inevitable edginess is entering the mind. All those 'what if' scenarios, and 'will I be able to handle it all again if something hasn't worked?' I don't want to think about it, but the mind's not listening.

'No more detours.'

I can't sleep, check-up day arrives, and yep, I'm a bag of nerves. And frankly for the first time in ages scared, really scared, just in case.......

'Please tell me everything's okay.' I'm praying as I meet Andrew again. He goes through the usual routine, but seems concerned that all is not as it should be.

'No, no, no, please not all that again.'

He explains 'the secondary in your neck hasn't reduced to the extent it should have done, so I'm concerned there may still be active cancer cells in there so you need to be re-scanned to check.'

'What are you saying' I blurt out, terrified 'please don't tell me I have to go through all that again.'

The picture of calm (he may have done this a few times before), he looks at me and starts. 'If the cells are alive I'll send you to John Timothy for surgery to have them cut out, and if they're dead, I'll recommend you go to John anyway to have any potentially infected glands/nodes removed. Everything else is absolutely fine'.

126

Slightly relieved I just reply 'get them out then, as I have no intention of being back here in a few months'. I am trying to sound confident, but inwardly feeling somewhat different. I leave unsure what to think. Down about needing more surgery, yet excellent about 'no further issues'.

The turmoil continues.

Underground

It's back to the world of basement scanners, men in white coats, valium, and radioactive glucose. Identical to before, but after the scan I notice a toilet with a large sign *'after scan use only'*.

'Why?' ask I.

'After scanning, your urine is so radioactive it would go through 'ordinary' porcelain in no time.' I was advised.

I left just pondering how could the body absorb so much punishment, on top of the chemo and radiotherapy, and still survive?

Now, **THE** meeting – what has this last scan shown up?

I went back to hospital with my stomach churning... *'what if the results showed something more? Try not to think about it.'*

And again, I can't help but wonder what this feels like from the other side. Maybe the consultant is stressed about running late – after all, he's got a family to get back to as well. He probably just wants to speed up and get finished, maybe grateful for an efficient secretary who has all the right notes ready for the next patient.

He must wonder, too, what it feels like from my side. He must have imagined himself in my shoes, wondering if the treatment has worked, empathising with this weird half-fearful, half-expectant state of mind.

'Hello Keith, you're looking better, how are you feeling? And are the taste and appetite returning as yet?'

'Getting better thanks, Andrew'. Today, I can't do small-talk and simply ask, 'what did the scan results show?' My hands are shaking nervously.

'Yes, they're in – those cancer cells in your neck are dead.'

I'm not sure what to feel. All the live cancer cells are gone. I should be ecstatic, but strangely it's more of a feeling of simple relief that I won't have to go through all this again.

'So you can go off on your trip to the Indian Ocean and relax.'

'Say that again – it just sounds so good!'

At last, at last, can't believe it! Get that factor 3000 sun cream (I absolutely must avoid sunburn on anywhere that's been subject to radiotherapy – no problem, I think I've had enough of cancer!)

No chance of a tan, but La Reunion, Madagascar, Sun City......here we come!

It's time to catch up with Mel and see how she's getting on.

'You sound happy' she says.

I update her with my news, and thankfully everything is progressing well with her (if not without discomfort), and we arrange our over-indulgent lunch for January.

Last lap

It's back into St. Anthony's one early afternoon in November, and the now familiar procedure. I'm shown the room, given a few hours to relax pre-op (ironic really, as it's somewhat tricky to relax knowing you are about to be 'put under' and cut open), and settle in.

Mads is with me, and John Timothy comes in to give me the low-down: 'I'm going to open up your neck at ear level, remove the secondary, go down the side of your neck and remove any other gland nearby, and sew you up again – you'll have an impressive scar!' he advises.

He continues: 'needless to say there are risks involved, the op being so close to shoulder muscles and the key nerves in your neck. The worst case scenario is one of those nerves is damaged, or severed, and the left side of the face could be paralysed.'

'Always so matter-of-fact when imparting what the worst-case scenarios could be'.

Obviously reading my thoughts, he smiled and stated confidently 'That's not going to happen, so no point in worrying about it. What is assured is some shoulder stiffness (any exercise will be a non-starter for the time being), and a numb bottom part of the jaw for the foreseeable future, or possibly ad infinitum. Also, you will have a scar a few inches long – as a memento of the last six months.'

No problems, next is the anaesthetist to cover how he'll put me under and then the porter will be round to wheel me off to the relevant op centre and wire me up.

Time for Mads to leave now just as I'm presented with my 'op gown'. Must look the part!

The porter arrives, a cheerful guy who's all smiles, and it's off to the anaesthetist, now dressed in his operating theatre 'uniform'. He wires me up, gives me a jab, tells me to put the oxygen mask on and breathe deeply.

The next thing I'm aware of is waking up in the recovery room and seeing John Timothy there, smiling. I have absolutely no memory at all of what he said in spite of apparently having a lengthy conversation.

Maybe the memory will be back tomorrow.

Finished!

Once I'm awake, and able to converse without forgetting everything immediately, I'm wheeled back to my room. Apparently the op lasted four hours, but all I'm aware of now is a tube coming out of my neck draining into a bottle, and heaven knows how many stitches in my neck. I have to say it's neatly done – almost a piece of art!

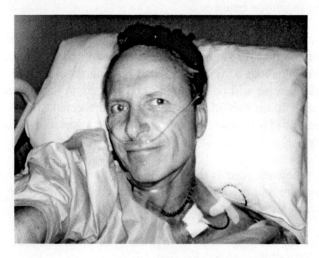

The final op.

Feeling awake now, it's a sandwich for dinner, one last check-up from the nurse and time for a sleep. One final adjustment required as I need to wear these rather fetching white skin-tight stockings – anti-DVT protection!

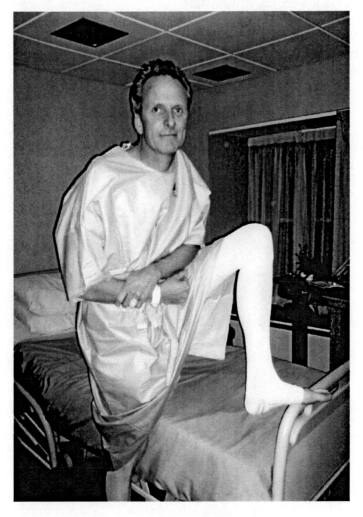

Anti DVT tights.

Get those legs! Never my best attribute!

Wake up the next morning feeling fine, and in absolutely no pain at all, which given that amount of sewing in my neck I'm amazed at. There's no sensation at all, a little strange as that tube is still 'inserted' in my neck – still, I suppose those painkillers are doing their stuff.

Mads is due in after breakfast, as is John Timothy, but the first visitor is the nurse who does the usual blood pressure and heart tests before checking 'the bottle' to see how much gunk has oozed out from the op overnight – she seems very pleased that there is so little.

It's all looking very promising now – the home stretch?

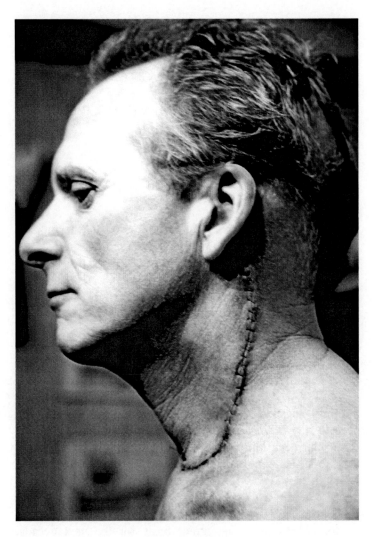

Neat handiwork.

The result

John arrives, casts an admiring look at his own handiwork
(on which I compliment him), before describing how it went.

133

He starts, 'the secondary tumour is now history as are all the lymph glands in that part of the neck.'

I can feel my heartbeat leap up now. *GO ON!*

'The op was 100% successful. You are CANCER FREE.'

Oh God, I've done it, at last!

I can feel myself start shaking in sheer relief. All those months of treatment, feeling dire, it's over!

No-one can possibly explain just how good that sounded. I just replay those words in my head over and over again, just thinking about what I've been through over the last few months.

I feel a huge grin spreading across my face *'Say that again, and again'*.

'Do you have any idea just how good that sounds?' I ask rather stupidly, as I suspect he has more than just an inkling!

Smiling, he adds: 'you're not quite done yet though, you need to stay in for a couple of days until nothing is draining from your neck into the bottle, but you should be 'released' very soon. He almost makes it sound like a prison sentence, which in an odd way I suppose it has been.

He continues: 'Now for what happens next. You will need to go for check-ups on a regular basis for the next decade. Starting monthly, these will alternate between myself and Andrew up at the Marsden. The first check-up will be ten days after you leave here, when the stitches will be removed. After six months these monthly check-ups will be dropped to every six weeks, after a year dropped to alternate months and so on.'

Finally he finishes his inspection and says I can get up and walk around, even go outside if I feel up to it, with which he turns and heads off with a cheerful 'see you in ten days'.

I'm left sitting there in bed with a huge smile: CANCER FREE! I've survived!

At last! CANCER FREE! CANCER FREE!

I reflect for a moment on one of John's comments about my first visit here.

During one of our conversations during this visit I had asked a question that had been intriguing me. 'So what would have happened if I wouldn't have found the small lump on my neck back in May? Or if the medics hadn't reacted immediately, as you said yourself it would extremely easy to miss the primary?'

'You would have been back here within three months, with a lump in your throat the size of a golf ball, probably coughing up blood, and well …'

Suffice to say my chances of making Christmas would have been minimal. It had been such a small lump, not causing me any problems.

I think I now understand the saying 'small, but deadly'.

I can't help but think how extremely fortunate I've been to be treated by such consummate professionals as Andrew and John, together with the fantastic back-up team of nurses, doctors, radiographers and all other hospital folk too numerous to list whom I've encountered during my many visits and stays in the various hospitals and medical centres I've been touring! A massive, massive thank you to all of them.

'Cancer free, cancer free'. Just how good does that sound?

Normal life

Mads arrives and I give her the news. A big hug, huge smiles and tears of relief rolling down our faces! We've been through rather a lot over the last six months, and the big trip is not far away now.

She just stares at the stitching in amazement at how neat it is, and is as stunned as I am that there is absolutely no pain. She stays for a while, we have a short stroll outside hand in hand (God I feel great now!), and then she leaves as I need rest, but will be back later with Jess.

Post-op day 1 is a mix of rest, eat, rest and watch TV with regular check-ups. It was mid-afternoon, about three o'clock when I had a surprise visitor, a nun dressed all in white. Never having met a nun before, I was a little unsure as to what to say, so opted for something trite like 'hello, how are you?' Anyway she was just stopping by to see how I was doing, as the hospital is linked to the Catholic Church.

Mads is back with Jess who also just stares at the stitching in my neck, but grabs the mobile to take some photos. Well trained!

I ask her to take some of the back of my head as well as I want to see the extent of my hair loss. There's virtually nothing left, no wonder I've been feeling the cold – all that radiotherapy had indeed left its mark.

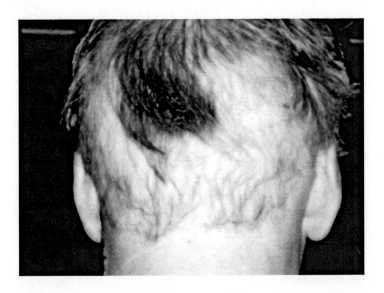

Radiotherapy side effect.

Mads and Jess leave knowing I'll be home within 48 hours. It's dinner time: looks like the roast pork this evening. I must say the food in here looks rather good.

'Wonder how long it will take before I can taste this properly.'

'Any chance of a glass of wine?' I enquire expecting a short, sharp response.

To my complete and utter surprise 'Yes' she replied, and produced a wine list. Was that a disapproving look? Who cares, and before I know it I have a half bottle of good red.

I just lie in bed, television on, sipping the wine, smiling, and replaying those words, 'YOU ARE CANCER FREE', over and over again. Probably the best four words I've ever heard. My own quiet celebration of the outcome!

Cheers, it's good to be alive......holidays soon!

Slap on the wrist

The last couple of days in hospital go fine. Mads and I go for a walk, out of the hospital, down the road, up the hill and back (the tube is still in my neck, and the draining bottle is neatly hidden away in my coat pocket), before returning, and the nurse drops by for the next check-up.

When I tell her where we've been I get the proverbial slap on the wrist as we've overdone the quiet stroll. 'That's way too far, what would've happened if you'd collapsed?' She ticked me off, perhaps a little tongue-in-cheek judging by her expression. Well, I hadn't collapsed, and it felt great to have gently pushed even the smallest of boundaries.

On the mend for sure.

It's over

John appears, takes one look and says it's fine to remove the tube and I can go home the next morning. Back home, it's late November and only two weeks until our holiday. My spirits are really high now.

Word is out about the re-appearance on the street of 'Frankenstein' so the neighbours are all curious about 'the scar'. Much amusement ensues when one suggested that if I had been 'released' a month earlier I'd have been sent out with the kids tricking and treating – no make-up required, just show them your stitches!

Back to hospital for the stitches removal, check-up and it's off home. I'm given a clean bill of health. The treatment really is done, finished, it's all over.

In many ways it does feel a little strange not to have any more medical treatment lined up. This, and all the resultant worries and general mental turmoil, have basically been my life for the last few months.

Now I can call the family and tell them all the 'official' news that I'm all clear. By now it's more of a relief to me than a cause for mass celebration, but to my family obviously rather more than that.

So, normal life can start to resume, give or take the odd check-up and ongoing side-effect or two.

The overall situation is looking great, just a couple of minor issues to work through in the short term. I've got very limited movement in my left shoulder after the last op. This is exactly as expected. I'm slightly surprised that no physio was recommended, but certainly happy to run with what I'm being advised (after all the advice has been faultless so far).

The recommendation is to re-start gentle exercise, particularly swimming and maybe some low-impact cardio work. Golf, real tennis and anything else strenuous is banned for the time being (next target on this front is, as ever, a holiday, this time skiing in Austria in February).

I've put back about half the weight I lost throughout radiotherapy, am now eating most things except spicy food (tomato ketchup doesn't rip my throat apart any more), but anything dry still needs glass after glass of water to get it down, and strangely fresh fruit tastes completely wrong.

All in all I'll take my current situation for sure!

Flying ducks

There is one more event to go before we're off. We are hosting the family Christmas, early in December, due to the holiday. This time Madeleine's parents are over from Sweden, so we will have to try them on the traditional

Christmas pudding – a token gesture to 'tradition' as we never do turkey anyway.

We start the traditional opening of presents and there's one from my brother-in-law, Pete, always to be viewed with a large degree of trepidation.

'Now what has he found this year?'

Over the past few years this has become something of a challenge – who can buy who the absolute 'naffest' present possible. This year I settled for a delightful blue 'ancient' Greek urn – I should perhaps point out this was his present a few years ago, but due to it being quite so ghastly has been passed back and forth ever since!

Pete had been working somewhat harder, scouring shops and markets all over and come up with his piece de resistance – a trio of flying ducks to nail to the wall. Bad enough so far it was about to get worse – with pride he carefully placed the largest on the wall above the front door and demonstrated how whenever it picked up a sound it dispensed a loud 'quack'.

I feel a bad accident coming on.

Sitting down to not-so-traditional dinner everyone raises their glass and says 'cheers' or 'skol' in Swedish. Mum then comments about how good it is that I'm still here and able to enjoy another Christmas – nice touch that brings a lump in my throat, so to speak!

Buffalo, steak or kudu?

It occurs to me that I had better just phone the travel insurance and inquire about my cover. Surprising result – not! if anything happens to me on the medical front that could possibly be related back to cancer I'm not covered.

Regardless, we're off, the first stop being one night in Johannesburg – we arrive at our hotel in time to check-in and wander off to get some lunch at the nearest shopping mall. We find a suitable-looking venue, and stop to admire the long list of meat dishes. Decisions, decisions, is it to be beefsteak? Maybe some buffalo? Or how about a slice or two of kudu?

South Africa is most definitely not a place for vegetarians – the steak that appeared was huge, and so tender it just melted in my mouth. What a great start to the holiday.

Mads happens to mention that Jess is looking a little swollen in the face. I reckon it's just the effect of the overnight flight, and am keen just to get on with enjoying the start of what will be a great trip for all. Inwardly I'm already panicking, praying this is not the re-appearance of her nephrotic syndrome, from which she had been cleared over two years ago.

Local customs

Off the next morning to catch the plane to Antananarivo for the connecting flight to La Reunion – 'lunch in Madagascar' has a rather classy ring to it.

We'd checked our bags straight through to La Reunion, so headed off to customs. They advised us we had to collect them, and in spite of our protestations that we're just transferring flights, we have to go back to the carousel.

Carousel empty! *'here goes, looks like the fun's about to begin'* I can't help feeling. The customs officers headed off in all directions to help, eventually finding the bags in a totally different part of the airport.

There is still plenty of coming and going to and from the customs desks, which is starting to cause some amusement.

Confusion reigned, but almost entirely due to my thirty year old 'O' level French being woefully inadequate to understand what on earth was happening. Once again Mads was able to apply her linguistic talent to help resolve the situation.

Eventually some helpful member of staff came, chatted, said he'd sort it out, relieved us of the luggage and passports and let us through to the restaurant.

It took a few seconds, but then…too late, he'd gone…

'What have we just done? He has all our luggage, connecting flight tickets, and passports!' Too late! We had just better hope he's honest!

Short on options we settled down in the restaurant, looking forward to 'airport haute cuisine' – omelette and chips times three with plenty of ketchup, and some very odd-tasting local Madagascan wine.

To our relief the customs man re-appeared in the restaurant with everything and we were off to La Reunion.

13 hours in a plane and land in France!

So after three flights, one night in Johannesburg and thirteen hours in a plane we landed on this volcanic island in the Indian Ocean, which is in France, where the currency is Euros and the language, not surprisingly, French. Weird feeling.

Anyway, we pick up the car and head off to the hotel. I chance a sideways look at Jess and she is definitely swollen in her face, the classic first signs of a relapse. Mads and I chat about her condition, and decide to see what happens over the next day, but by the following evening it's not changed so Mads says go to the doctors.

I'm reluctant to accept this as I can see the end of the trip before it's started, but in the long-run we must sort it out. As Mads says we're better off going to the doctors in France than in Madagascar so let's go – no doctors around so let's try the hospital.

The back entrance to A&E is fine, and the staff couldn't have been more helpful. Communication was interesting: a mixture of their few English words with our limited French and we kind of understood.

The outcome was, unfortunately, all too predictable. She had indeed had a relapse into nephrotic syndrome, so heavy duty steroids it will be (luckily they use the same prednisolone tablets over here that Jess has had previously).

The other news wasn't so good. 'You can't go on to Madagascar as there are no decent medical facilities there, and really she shouldn't be in the sunshine' the doctor duly informed us. There it was, the final blow to the holiday.

That's it then, the trip's over, before it's really started. It's Mads I feel most for as she really needed some time to chill out and relax after the strains of the last few months, but it isn't to be.

Fully insured?

Time to call travel insurance and get moving – to say they were not entirely helpful would be an understatement.

We spent god knows how long following overly-complicated insurance 'requirements' on various phone calls to Kingston Hospital (where Jess had been previously treated), the GP back home, in order to get all the medical information required by the travel insurance policy. Or more precisely, the Copenhagen-based call centre of the first company involved, who handle any incidents for another insurance company, on a policy which appears on yet another company's letterhead but is still somehow one travel insurance policy.

Work that one out if you can, but it is guaranteed to confuse, frustrate and generally delay any speedy handling of the situation.

Once they found out that Jess had suffered from this before, their attitude hardened, and they went straight down the track of 'it's a pre-existing condition that you hadn't told us about therefore it wasn't covered'. Eventually, after another round of numerous international phone calls all the documents had been located, and they finally admitted that it had been mentioned correctly previously, was on the correct documents, and the 'all clear' had been documented previously.

I have no idea what the phone bill will be, but long calls from the depths of the Indian Ocean aren't cheap, and let me guess, that is a cost that won't be covered in the policy.

It all takes so long to sort out that we need to extend our five night stay in La Reunion, and in spite of everything we manage to have a good few days as it's a fantastic island.

Mads and I go on the most hair-raising flight ever – a couple of hours up and around the centre of the island (over 10,000 feet high) in an over-sized microlite.

Or, more accurately, a seat attached to a couple of metal bars, wrapped in canvas-type material with a small engine and a propeller. Oh and thankfully a pilot!

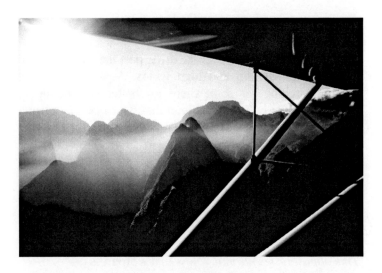

Amazing experience!

It was fantastic fun until it hit the turbulence – suddenly it became rather like what I would imagine being in a pea in a food processor when it's turned on! and only a few thousand feet up.

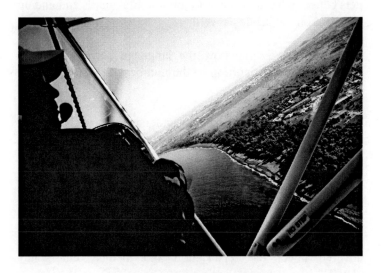

'This is your captain speaking'.

French food

Just for good measure a cyclone drifts past the island and we get the torrential rain and high winds. At least the rain's warm! Searching for somewhere to shelter we end up in seemingly the only local restaurant that stays open, and being in France (it still seems strange that we've flown for 13 hours in three separate flights and are in France) the food is excellent.

With a restricted menu due to the cyclone, we order the local 'catch of the day' which turns out to be a delicious local white fish.

'This almost tastes normal.' Now that's progress.

We start chatting with a bunch of lifeguards who are in party mood – they've got the night off.

The rain is lashing down now, the wind howling, but it's still lovely and warm. The lights go out. Power's down! It's looking like a very entertaining evening in the wet, and just gets better as we are invited to join the life guards and end up very wet on the inside as well!

It always amazes me how the language barriers seem to reduce in direct proportion to the number of glasses of wine consumed.

Soon we are having no trouble understanding each other at all, not that I have any idea what we talked about.

Insurance nightmare

We finally get the travel insurance sorted, but they drop into the conversation 'only your daughter and one of you are covered under the repatriation and medical emergency clause'.

'WHAT?' , just about managing to hold back saying what I really want to, and continue, with the merest hint of sarcasm 'so the other is supposed to continue with the holiday as though nothing has happened, knowing that our daughter is going home early because of a medical emergency – do you think that's reasonable?'

This is a question that I asked numerous times, but unsurprisingly was never answered, on each occasion being met with the 'company line'. 'Sorry, that's what the policy says'. So once again insurance small-print seemingly ensures that the cover is not as complete as would have been expected.

To say we're livid would be an understatement, and any thoughts of at least some relaxation disappear as stress levels have risen alarmingly. We have no option but to shell out £1,500 for a one–way ticket home.

I should point out that this is a policy on which all three of us are named, therefore one would think 'covered', and the medical emergency and repatriation clause provides cover for up to £10 million, at least that what the front page of the policy states. Typical insurance: just when you need it most, the company can be relied upon to find some unreasonable piece of small-print, or some excuse that means the claim will not be settled in the expected manner.

Most importantly, however, we need to get home so Jess can get the treatment she needs, and we'll take this up later. Six months down track (and after at least two letters of complaint, and numerous phone calls) the insurance company finally accepted that the other return flight should be covered, but only under the 'holiday curtailment' clause (rather than the repatriation clause), and only if we can provide the third boarding pass to prove we were on the flight.

'That'll be the flight that you booked two of us onto then?' I can't help mentioning.

A tough year

So our three week Christmas/new Year wonder trip now gets us back to not-so-sunny Thames Ditton mid-afternoon on Christmas Eve. 'The street' are aware of the situation as Jess has been on the internet in La Reunion – as she couldn't go in the sunshine then it was a pretty good way of her passing the time of day.

Within half an hour of getting home we've had three offers of "come and join us for Christmas dinner". What a fantastic street we live in. Thanking all profusely we've already decided we'll turn up unannounced at my parents.

When we arrive there's a mixture of stunned looks, and the over-riding sensation that my parents are delighted we have appeared! So turkey and Christmas pud it is then – 26 hours on a plane is the furthest I've travelled to get traditional Christmas dinner, but eat the lot, and taste most of it. It's not back to normal yet, but definitely improving.

There is a feeling that our luck really is due for a change for the better. As if 2007 hadn't had enough bad news, this holiday termination felt like one more kick in the teeth from a year that had delivered a few too many already.

Back home in Thames Ditton after a couple of days with the family, and we'll be there for the annual New Years' Eve street party, who knows we may even end up hosting it! This year it transpires it's not our turn.

At midnight Mads and I raise a glass, look at each other and drink one last

'Good riddance to 2007 that was one hell of a year, bring on 2008. '

148

More hospitals

It's back into the hospital routine again, into Kingston Hospital with Jess. They know us well as she's been in twice for nephrotic syndrome, once for the appendix last year, not to mention nearly dying from meningitis as a baby. It appears that all is on track as we know what the routine is, and once again are left hoping this is the last relapse.

As for me, it's back into the Marsden for the latest check-up with Andrew Jones. I'm a little nervous about this one. Stress is one of those things best avoided with cancer, and there's been plenty of it the last few weeks, courtesy of the travel insurance world.

'Good Christmas holiday?' Andrew asks.

Not quite sure where to start, but opt for a casual 'could have been better'.

He comments on how well I look, which is great to hear, and I explain that the taste is improving all the time, but I still have a dry mouth and need loads of water but that's a minor issue really.

'That's as expected' he says nonchalantly – very reassuring to hear as I settle back to 'enjoy' the now familiar look around the mouth, the feel of the neck and then that still strange sensation of the 'camera on a tube' being gently eased up one nostril, up my nose and down the back of my throat to check the old primary site.

'Excellent, you're doing fantastically well' he concludes.

Great news: and it occurs to me that what with one thing and another, I haven't really thought much about my situation in the last couple of weeks.

It's great to hear everything's moving ahead nicely, and with Jess on the mend too, the holiday disaster is rapidly becoming just a bad memory.

I've also caught up with a couple of 'cancer contacts' now. I've exchanged emails with the nurse, Kim, about meeting up and discussing the wedding photography I'm going to do. I really want to deliver a fantastic set of shots for her, after what she did for me hospital. July now doesn't seem that far away!

It's also good to be back arranging some more photographic work

That over-indulgent lunch

I've finally spoken to Mel who works down the road in Kingston, and arranged our much-discussed lunch in Thames Ditton. It's fantastic to see her again, looking so good with that radiant smile of hers, and we swap stories about treatment, side effects, recovery, people and their attitudes, taste, dry mouth and so on.

We hadn't seen each other since my last radiotherapy session, nearly four months ago – and then in that none-too-cheerful queue in the depths of the Royal Marsden Hospital.

Now for lunch – first up something to drink – most importantly a litre of water, and a bottle of red for strictly medicinal purposes of course!

'What would you like to eat?' I ask.

'What's got the most sauce, won't be spicy, and is likely to be the easiest dish to chew?' Funny how menu selection is now so different to those pre-cancer days.

We laugh spontaneously as it's probably the first time either of us has ever been browsing a menu knowing exactly what the other one is thinking, and with exactly the same limitations to diet.

Mel selects a gravy-heavy stew, but for me – well it has to be 'bangers and mash'. My first mouthful of solid food back in September, it was a non-decision.

Another bottle of wine, some dessert, and we stumble back home to say hi to the family – this is the first time Mel has met Mads and Jess. They are fascinated to meet her having heard all my stories.

Wry smiles all round as it's 'a little' obvious we've had a glass or two too many, but that was always going happen.

Mel had even arranged for one of her work mates to come and be her chauffeur service.

Fabulous lunch – so good to see her again.

Looking forward

It's time for my first check-up of 2008 – these are every two weeks to start with, alternating between the Anthony's, where I had the surgery, and The Royal Marsden where I had all the chemo and radio treatment.

'You can start gentle exercise again, but be mindful of the op on your neck, and how it will affect your shoulder', John Timothy tells me.

It's off to join the gym, along with all those new members who've made rash resolutions as Big Ben strikes to bring the new year in – *'how many will still be doing it in three weeks?'* I wonder.

In the back of my mind I have an idea I would like to do one of those treks as a fund-raiser. I'd seen some adverts on the wall in the Royal Marsden, and ponder on the fact that the only reason I am still here is the medical research that has enabled cancer treatment to be so effective, and the people that so ably administered it.

I would like to give something back. I guess my way of saying thanks for saving my life. Remember to ask at the next check-up when a reasonable timescale would be for this.

Also, I need to get the business moving again. It is now months since I have done any work, and consequently not earned a penny. Thank God for Mads' job, but it would be great to get the work coming in again. Besides which, I just enjoy the photography.

Next target

Needless to say: a holiday. The aim now is to get at least a little fitter as in a few weeks we are off on an eight day skiing trip to our favourite resort, Saalbach/Hinterglemm in Austria.

The early February check-up is here, and John goes through the normal check-list – all going really well. 'What about the shoulder and skiing?' I ask.

He takes a deep breath, looks me straight in the eyes and says calmly 'Don't know about that, it's a little soon'. I have a hunch he's winding me up, or by now just knows how I think.

Just before I show too much disappointment he smiles, 'you have more movement in your shoulder than the vast majority who've had similar surgery, and providing you're careful it'll be fine'.

'Careful? On skis? Me? If only I had that degree of control'. Bereft of much in the way of style and technique I somehow manage to get down most slopes, even if these days it's a bit slow for Jess.

The best news is at the end of the session. Subject to the next check-up being okay as well I'll be put back to six-weekly visits from the present monthly. I leave here with spring in the step, and it's Austria here we come.

Alpine diet

Skiing trips are nothing like they were twenty years ago. Then it was up on the mountain at 8 a.m., let's do the mountain before lunch, another this afternoon, and copious amounts of the apres ski. Or at least, that's the way it seems, with the benefit of hindsight!

These days it's all much more leisurely – or should that be middle-aged? We ease ourselves gently onto the mountain by around 9.30/10(ish), a couple of warm-up slopes, quick coffee and schnapps, and head off with regular stops to take in the scenery and avoid dehydration.

'Oh not another stop, can't we keep going?' has become Jess' plaintive cry as we nip in for a coffee here, a gluhwein there. This is the first year she's the one at the bottom first, asking why I'm so slow, and can't we do something steeper. 'Go and ask Mum if you want the icy black runs, and I'll meet you at the bottom!'

'Wurst and chips, spaghetti bolognaise, platters of ham and cheese – good wholesome mountain food, washed down with a beer, makes for an excellent midday break, although not necessarily making it easier to get skiing in the afternoon! I firmly believe all the serious skiing should be pre-lunch, just leaving a leisurely cruising slope or two for afterwards.

We've been back here a few times now, and given there are so many good restaurants just hidden away off the piste I keep thinking about writing the 'discerning mountain restaurant guide' with a photo or two - maybe next year.

I manage to ski all eight days which is an unexpected bonus, and return home to look forward to an excellent year of travel. Weekends in Bruges/Lille, New York and Portugal in the next month or so, an eleven day photo tour of Morocco, then later in the year two trips to Tuscany, France and Christmas in Florida...all looking terrific.

And the photography is starting to pick up and get busy again, I'm now nearly back to where I was before being diagnosed last year...... onwards and upwards.

The only one area not totally back to normal is taste – I still can't manage anything spicy as the throat is too sensitive...who knows if this will come back.

Just how much did *'that'* phone call in May last year change my life?

Closing thought

How lucky am I to have a second chance at life, and I don't intend to waste it!

9. Thanks

I can't finish this without a massive thank you to all those who have helped me pull through, in no particular order:

- To my family for all their strength and support – Mads and Jess at home: god knows what stress you've been under but just thanks for being there. Anna for the taxi service when most required, the hospital photography, and the first proof-read of this! Jane, Anna, my parents, Rick, Pete and Madeleine's family in Sweden for the ongoing encouragement and support.

- To the GP and doctors for referring me at the start - if you find a lump anywhere and are unsure what it is, get it checked out by the medics. It might just save your life!

- To Helen – for helping me to keep the mental part in the right place, and coming up with the idea of keeping a photo diary. I have had the chance to at least promote her services on an LBC radio phone-in on cancer. Helen, you know if you ever need a reference no matter what time of day or night just call it would be a pleasure!

- To friends – new and old: old - for your support and polite 'you're looking great' when I now know I must have looked like the walking dead! New: that's you Mel. Thanks for being so cheerful when I was at my lowest in those radiotherapy sessions, I just hope I managed to cheer you up in a similar manner to how you helped me. And it's just great to compare notes during those over-indulgent lunches!

- Tom 'The Bookwright', Malcolm, Anna, Rick, Mads, Tim and all the others who have helped me get this book together in a publishable form.

- Lesley for suggesting MX Publishing, and Steve for taking the book on.

- Last, but absolutely not least to all the medical staff - what total, utter and complete stars all of you are. Quite simply I just don't know how you do it, but will be eternally grateful you manage to see past the less pleasant sights and sounds of cancer wards, and continue treating, cajoling, encouraging (even if some gentle bullying is needed occasionally) us patients to recover when there must be plenty of times when that's not easy!

10. Postscript

It's now September 2009, over two years since diagnosis, and some twenty one months since the all clear. So where am I now?

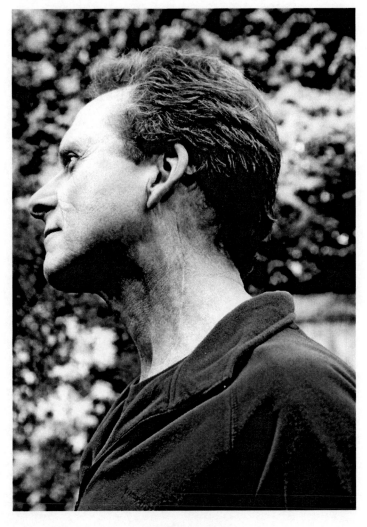

Small memento.

Health: my check-ups are progressing very well and have just been put back to quarterly.

Side-effects: appetite and taste are back as was. I still have a slightly dry mouth, but that's receding steadily, and not a problem. The taste for spicy food returned all of a sudden last summer, but it looks like the madras curry and Thai tom yum soups may be off for longer. The biggest side-effect is how much more I feel the cold now.

Appearance: my weight is steady, back to within a few pounds of when it all began. The hair on the back of my head grew back months ago albeit slightly darker.

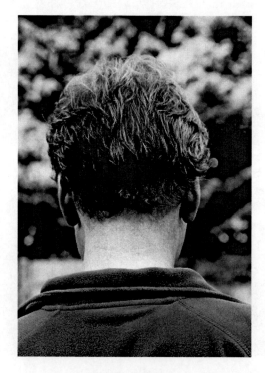

Back to normal.

Travel – as ever I am looking to get away as often as possible…. We did go back to Saalbach/Hinterglemm in February (and the restaurant guide is now complete in draft form), a weekend in Guernsey in April , weekend golfing in Norway in June, Tuscany in July and again in November, the trek in Iceland in August, and a late year trip to Kuala Lumpur, Bali and Lombok. Mads will get her r&r in the sunshine, even if it's two years later than planned!

The 'big one' – Mads and I are planning the ultimate celebration when I get to five years cancer clear. The plan is to rent the house out for a year and 'go' – spend a year going overland from the top of Canada to the bottom of Chile and round into Argentina.

Photography – I did shoot Kim's wedding last summer - hope she liked the results! After the 'time out' in 2007/2008, the business is back to pre-cancer levels, I have also won half a dozen photo awards in the US in 2008, and in April 2009 won a local photo competition in Kingston, on the theme of 'Beauty: inside and out''. Plus there may even be some business opportunities arising from the shots taken on the Iceland trek.

Travel insurance – after seven months the insurance company finally acknowledged that the other flight should have been covered and paid up, but only under a different clause. As an aside, I have discovered that it seems to be insurance industry practice to only cover one parent under the repatriation clause, but most seem to cover the other under 'curtailment' however you will have to stand your ground and fight very hard to get the refund. I wonder how much money the insured miss out on due to this situation – I suspect rather a lot!

Family – all well, and looking forward to a hospital-free time.

Learning Italian – watch out you guys at 'La Vecchia Banana' in Pondetera we'll be back with 'buonasera, una bottiglia di vino rosso di casa per favore'..... I have to admit my enthusiasm waned and I stopped the lessons in summer 2008, but Mads is still going well picking up her umpteenth language.

Fundraising – I never forgot seeing that leaflet I saw whilst in hospital, and in August 2009 completed the Iceland trek, which was quite simply one of the most unforgettable experiences of my life.

Thirty five complete strangers met at Heathrow and headed off to fundraise, each for their own chosen cause, and we were taken way outside any comfort zones on the trek through this stunning country. If any of you trekkers are reading this thanks for the company, the memories, it was an awesome trip, and we did it! Needless to say it wouldn't have worked without our team of experts leading us through the wilderness so thanks to you guys too.

At the time of writing I have raised over £6,200 for The Royal Marsden Cancer Charity and still hope to get up to £7,000. I ended up being the top fundraiser on the trek.

Just enough time and space to slip in a few shots from that most memorable experience.

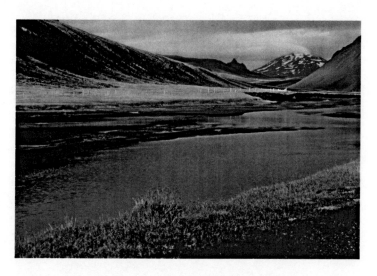

Morning view from near the first campsite.

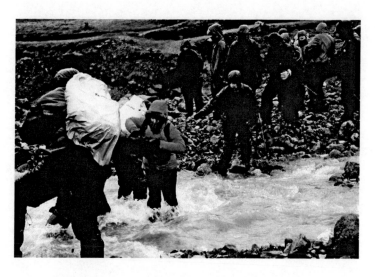

Wading through freezing melt-water channels.

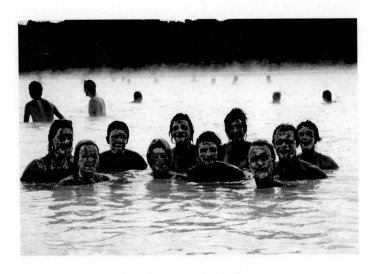

Face packs at The Blue Lagoon.

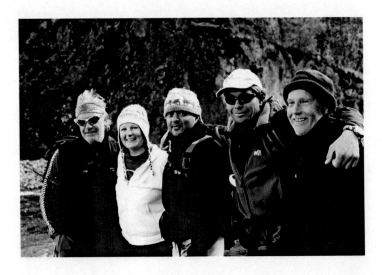

The experts.

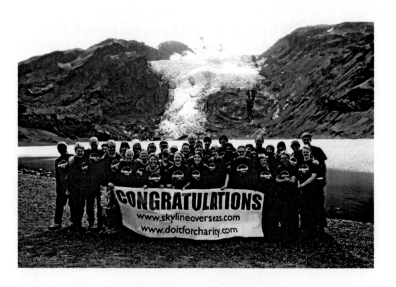

The trekking fundraisers.

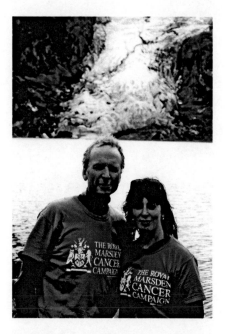

Fundraisers for The Royal Marsden.

To me the trek represented a huge personal triumph given when I first saw the leaflet in summer 2007 I didn't know if I would live to see 2008.

It's great to be alive!

NB – all the names of the consultants, doctors, nurses and any other of the superb medical staff I encountered have been changed – I would just like to say one final, massive THANKS to you all! Without you I wouldn't be here..........

Terminology

There are quite a few medical terms used in my story, so hopefully the following will help to explain what some of them actually mean, in a non-technical sort of way:

MRI scan   - full body scan in a magnetic tube that takes numerous cross-sectional images of the body to locate any tumours. (MRI is Magnetic Resonance Imaging).

CT (or CAT) scan - takes a series of x-ray images which help determine the exact site and size of any tumour. (CT is computerised tomography, CAT computerised axial tomography).

PET scan   - this uses radioactive tracers (glucose in my case) which then react with any cancer cells, so shows how many tumours exist. (PET is Positon Emission Tomography)

Squamous cell cancer – the type of cancer I had, and apparently 90% of all head and neck cancers are this type.

Cisplatin and 5FU - the two chemotherapy drugs that I was treated with.

EDTA   - pre-chemo tests carried on kidney functionality to check the kidneys are able to take the chemo drugs.

Other Resources

Self-hypnosis CDs and others are available from www.suzismith.net

Additional information on coaching and NLP at www.helenoakwater.co.uk

Also from MX Publishing

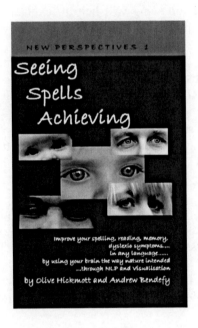

Seeing Spells Achieving

The UK's leading NLP book for
learning difficulties including dyslexia

More NLP books at www.mxpublishing.co.uk

Also from MX Publishing

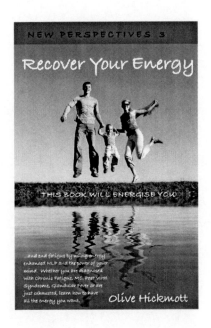

Recover Your Energy

NLP for Chronic Fatigue, ME and tiredness

More NLP books at www.mxpublishing.co.uk

Lightning Source UK Ltd.
Milton Keynes UK
171152UK00001B/54/P